Embrace Wellness and Radiate Confidence From The Inside Out

HER HEALTHY
Glow

HANNA OLIVAS & ADRIANA LUNA CARLOS
Along With 14 Inspiring Authors

TABLE OF CONTENTS

INTRODUCTION

Welcome to *Her Healthy Glow: Embrace Wellness and Radiate Confidence From the Inside Out*.

In a world that often focuses on external beauty and quick fixes, this book offers a refreshing and empowering perspective—true radiance comes from within. When you nourish your body, mind, and spirit, you unlock a glow that transcends superficial appearances, creating a lasting sense of well-being and confidence that shines from the inside out.

This guide is more than just a wellness book—it's a journey toward rediscovering your inner strength, vitality, and self-love. Through practical strategies, inspiring stories, and expert advice, you'll learn how to balance all aspects of your life, from physical health to mental clarity, and emotional resilience.

You'll explore holistic practices that nourish and rejuvenate, along with simple yet transformative habits to help you embrace each day with a renewed sense of purpose and positivity. This book will inspire you to cultivate a lifestyle that reflects the vibrant, radiant version of yourself that you were always meant to be.

Her Healthy Glow invites you to step into your power, embrace your wellness journey, and radiate confidence like never before. The path to a healthier, more vibrant you starts here—let's begin this transformation together.

Ready to glow? Let's dive in!

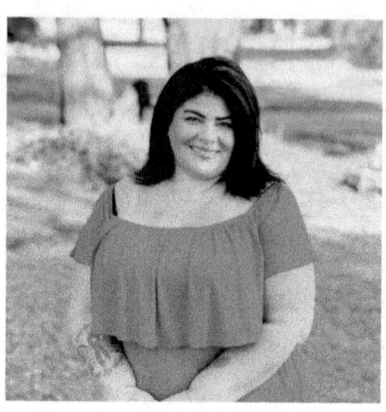

Hanna Olivas

Founder and CEO of SHE RISES STUDIOS

https://www.linkedin.com/company/she-rises-studios/
https://www.facebook.com/sherisesstudios
https://www.instagram.com/sherisesstudios_llc/
www.SheRisesStudios.com

Author, Speaker, and Founder. Hanna was born and raised in Las Vegas, Nevada, and has paved her way to becoming one of the most influential women of 2022. Hanna is the co-founder of She Rises Studios and the founder of the Brave & Beautiful Blood Cancer Foundation. Her journey started in 2017 when she was first diagnosed with Multiple Myeloma, an incurable blood cancer. Now more than ever, her focus is to empower other women to become leaders because The Future is Female. She is currently traveling and speaking publicly to women to educate them on entrepreneurship, leadership, and owning the female power within.

The Healthy Glow:
Unleashing the Radiance Within

By Hanna Olivas

In a world where external appearances often overshadow the essence of true beauty, the concept of a "healthy glow" transcends mere physical attributes. It is a powerful manifestation of a woman's vitality, self-love, and inner strength. It's that ethereal quality that radiates from someone who embraces her whole being—mind, body, and spirit. This glow isn't just about the clarity of our skin or the brightness of our eyes; it embodies the deep connection we forge with ourselves and the world around us.

To have a healthy glow is to feel vibrant and alive, to be in tune with the rhythms of life, and to exude joy and confidence. It's a state of being where physical health and emotional well-being intertwine, creating a beautiful harmony that shines through in every aspect of life. This glow is a beacon of resilience and authenticity, illuminating the path for others as we navigate life's challenges and triumphs.

"Your glow is not just a reflection of your outer beauty; it is a testament to your journey, your strength, and your resilience."

Understanding the Importance of a Healthy Glow

The journey to achieving a healthy glow is a personal one, deeply rooted in self-love and self-care. For many women, it often begins with a pivotal moment of realization—an awakening to the fact that we deserve to prioritize our health and well-being. This journey is not just about aesthetics; it is about nurturing our souls, healing from past wounds, and embracing our authentic selves.

In a society that bombards us with images of perfection, we often find ourselves chasing unrealistic standards. However, true beauty is not defined by filters or the number on a scale. It is a deep-rooted self-acceptance that flourishes when we choose to honor our unique journeys. Embracing our flaws, celebrating our victories, and learning from our struggles is what cultivates a glow that is both genuine and enduring.

Nourishing Your Body

Nourishing our bodies is a fundamental step on the path to achieving that radiant glow. What we feed ourselves has a profound impact on our physical and emotional health. A well-balanced diet rich in fruits, vegetables, whole grains, and healthy fats fuels our bodies and enhances our vitality. The importance of hydration cannot be overstated; water is a vital elixir that maintains skin elasticity and overall health.

However, nourishment is not solely about restrictive diets or calorie counting. It involves developing a healthy relationship with food—one that is grounded in love and respect rather than guilt and shame. It's essential to allow ourselves to indulge in our favorite foods while also being mindful of what we consume. It's about celebrating food as a source of nourishment and joy rather than viewing it as a battleground for self-discipline.

"Food is not just fuel; it is a source of nourishment and joy. Let it be a celebration of life."

I vividly recall my own journey with food. There was a time when I would obsessively count calories and scrutinize every bite. It felt like a never-ending battle against my own body. But as I began to embrace a more holistic approach, everything changed. I learned to listen to my body's cues and trust its wisdom. Instead of depriving myself, I started to explore new flavors and nourish my body with the foods it craved. This shift not only transformed my physical health but also liberated my spirit.

Embracing Movement

Movement is another essential component of cultivating a healthy glow. Physical activity is not just about shedding pounds or fitting into a certain size; it is about celebrating our bodies and their capabilities. Exercise releases endorphins, elevating our mood and alleviating stress. The key is to find a form of movement that resonates with you—whether it's dancing, hiking, yoga, or simply taking a brisk walk in nature.

I remember the first time I stepped onto a yoga mat. It was a humble beginning, filled with awkward poses and a racing mind. Yet, as I continued to practice, I found solace in the stillness. Each session became a sacred space where I could reconnect with myself, breathe deeply, and let go of the chaos of life. The feeling of flowing through poses, anchored in my breath, ignited a spark within me. I began to realize that movement is an act of self-love, an offering to my body that honors its strength and grace.

Prioritizing Mental Health

Mental health is an integral part of our overall well-being. In a world that often overlooks the importance of emotional wellness, it's crucial for women to prioritize their mental health just as much as their physical health. Engaging in mindfulness practices, such as meditation, journaling, or simply taking a moment to breathe deeply, can help clear mental clutter and create space for positivity and gratitude.

During the toughest times in my life, I turned to journaling as a means of release. Penning down my thoughts and feelings became a therapeutic outlet. It was in those pages that I confronted my fears, processed my pain, and celebrated my victories. I discovered that writing not only served as a tool for reflection but also as a bridge to self-discovery. Each entry was a testament to my resilience and a reminder of the power I held within.

Seeking support from friends, family, or professionals is equally essential. We are not meant to navigate life's challenges alone, and opening up about our struggles can foster deeper connections with others. When we create safe spaces for vulnerability, we allow ourselves to heal and grow. The act of sharing our burdens can lighten the load and build a sense of community and understanding.

"Your vulnerability is not a weakness; it is a testament to your strength and a source of connection."

Cultivating a Supportive Community

Women possess an incredible ability to lift each other up. When we come together, we create an environment where everyone can thrive. Supporting one another means celebrating each other's successes, offering a listening ear, and providing encouragement during difficult times. It is in these moments of connection that we find strength and empowerment.

Imagine a circle of women, each glowing with their unique light, sharing their journeys, and inspiring one another. This sense of community is vital for nurturing our healthy glow. We should strive to create spaces where we can share our stories, learn from one another, and inspire collective growth.

"When women come together, magic happens. Together, we can rise, shine, and unleash our collective power."

In my own life, I have been fortunate to find a tribe of incredible women who support and uplift one another. Whether it's through weekly coffee dates, virtual gatherings, or simply sending a text to check in, these connections have been lifelines. The beauty of shared experiences—celebrating milestones, offering a shoulder to cry on, or cheering each other on—has illuminated my path and reminded me that I am never alone.

The Power of Self-Love

At the core of the healthy glow is self-love. This means embracing ourselves as we are—flaws, scars, and all. It requires us to recognize our worth and appreciate our unique beauty. Self-love is not a destination; it is an ongoing practice that involves compassion, understanding, and forgiveness.

Learning to love ourselves can be challenging, especially for those who have experienced trauma or pain. For years, I battled with feelings of unworthiness, stemming from past experiences that left scars on my heart. It wasn't until I embarked on a journey of self-discovery that I realized the importance of treating myself with the same kindness I extended to others. I began to replace negative self-talk with affirmations of love and appreciation. I celebrated my strengths while acknowledging my weaknesses, understanding that both are integral parts of who I am.

"You are worthy of love, joy, and all the beautiful things life has to offer. Embrace your worthiness."

Keeping the Glow Alive Through Life's Challenges

Life is an unpredictable journey filled with ups and downs. We all face challenges, trauma, and heartache that can dim our glow. However, it is possible to keep that glow alive even in the face of adversity.

First and foremost, allow yourself to feel. It's okay to grieve, to be angry, or to feel lost. These emotions are part of the human experience, and acknowledging them is essential for healing. By giving ourselves permission to feel, we can move through pain rather than burying it.

Engaging in self-care practices during difficult times is vital. Whether through journaling, connecting with nature, or simply taking a moment to breathe deeply, self-care serves as a reminder that we deserve love and attention, even when life feels overwhelming. When I found myself grappling with overwhelming sadness, I turned to nature as my refuge. Long walks in the park, the rustle of leaves, and the soft whispers of the wind became my solace. Nature has a remarkable ability to ground us and remind us of the beauty that exists in the world, even amidst chaos.

"In the depths of despair, remember to breathe. In every breath lies the power to reclaim your glow."

Additionally, cultivating resilience can help us navigate challenges with grace. Resilience is not about being unbreakable; it's about embracing our vulnerabilities and learning to rise again. Each setback can serve as a lesson, and each struggle can contribute to our growth.

"Resilience is not the absence of struggle; it is the courage to rise again and shine even brighter."

I often reflect on the times in my life when I faced seemingly insurmountable challenges. Each experience taught me valuable lessons about perseverance and strength. It was through those trials that I discovered the depths of my resilience and the power of hope. I learned that while life may knock us down, it also grants us the strength to rise again, even stronger than before.

The Essence of the Healthy Glow

So, what does the healthy glow look and feel like? It's the sparkle in a woman's eyes when she's fully present in the moment, embracing the beauty of life with all its imperfections. It's the warmth that radiates from a smile that is genuine and unforced, reflecting a heart at peace with itself. It's the vibrant energy that emanates from someone who has learned to honor her journey, to love herself fiercely, and to rise above the challenges life throws her way.

A woman with a healthy glow embodies confidence and authenticity. She knows her worth, and she is not afraid to shine her light. This glow doesn't fade in the face of adversity; instead, it deepens as she navigates through life's complexities with grace and strength. The glow is amplified by the connections she forges with others, the love she shares, and the compassion she extends to herself and those around her.

In our journey to maintain this glow, it is crucial to recognize that it is not a constant state. Life is filled with ebbs and flows, and our glow may dim at times due to stress, heartbreak, or loss. However, it is essential to understand that we can always return to our glow. It is a part of us, deeply rooted in our essence. It may take time and effort to rekindle, but it is always there, waiting to be reignited.

Creating a Ritual of Self-Care

Establishing a ritual of self-care is one way to keep the healthy glow alive. This ritual can be as simple or elaborate as you wish. It could involve setting aside a few minutes each day to meditate, taking a long bath filled with soothing oils, or spending time in nature to recharge. Whatever form it takes, the key is to create a sacred space where you can reconnect with yourself.

In my own life, I have found that morning rituals are particularly powerful. The quiet moments before the world awakens provide an opportunity to set intentions for the day ahead. I take time to breathe deeply, express gratitude, and envision the kind of energy I want to carry with me. This simple practice centers me and serves as a reminder of my worth and the importance of nurturing my well-being.

"In the stillness of the morning, I find my strength. It is here that I remind myself of my purpose and the beauty that resides within me."

The Collective Power of Women

As we embrace our own healthy glow, let us not forget the power of lifting one another. In a world that often pits women against each other, it is vital to foster a sense of community and sisterhood. When women support one another, we create a ripple effect of empowerment that can change lives. Each time we cheer for another woman's success or offer a helping hand during difficult times, we contribute to a culture of compassion and understanding.

Imagine a world where women celebrate each other's achievements without jealousy or comparison. This world is within reach, but it requires a conscious effort to uplift those around us. Let us challenge ourselves to be the source of positivity in each other's lives. By sharing our stories, our struggles, and our triumphs, we pave the way for future generations of women to shine unapologetically.

"When we rise together, we create a legacy of strength and beauty that echoes through time."

Conclusion: Embracing Your Healthy Glow

In conclusion, the journey to discovering and nurturing your healthy glow is a deeply personal and transformative process. It requires us to embrace self-love, prioritize our well-being, and foster connections with others. It is about recognizing our worth and allowing ourselves to shine brightly, even in the face of adversity.

As you embark on this journey, remember that the glow is not a destination; it is a continuous journey of growth and self-discovery. Embrace the beautiful imperfections that make you uniquely you, and never underestimate the power of your light. When you shine, you not only illuminate your path but also inspire others to embrace their own radiance.

"You are a masterpiece in progress, and your glow is a testament to the incredible journey that is uniquely yours."

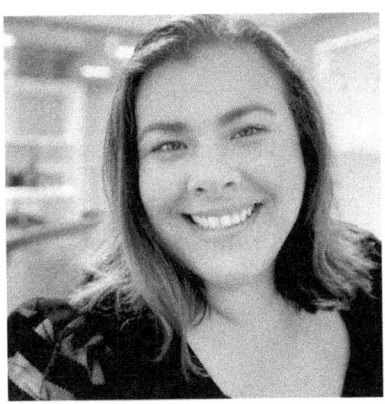

Adriana Luna Carlos

Founder and CEO of SHE RISES STUDIOS & FENIX TV

https://www.linkedin.com/in/adriana-luna-carlos/
https://www.facebook.com/adrianalunacarlos
https://www.instagram.com/sherisesstudios_llc/
https://www.sherisesstudios.com/
https://fenixtv.app/

Adriana Luna Carlos is an accomplished web and graphic designer, author, and mentor with a passion for helping women succeed in life and business. With over 10 years of experience in graphic and web arts, Adriana has built a reputation as an innovative leader and entrepreneur. In 2020, she co-founded She Rises Studios, a multi-digital media company and publishing house that has helped countless clients achieve their branding and marketing goals. In 2023, she co-created FENIX TV, an online streaming platform that showcases stories of people breaking barriers, shattering stereotypes, and triumphing against the odds.

As an advocate for women's success, Adriana challenges her clients and mentees to strive for nothing less than excellence. She has a deep understanding of the insecurities and challenges that women often face in the business world and provides the guidance and resources needed to overcome them. Her success as a business leader and entrepreneur has made her a sought-after mentor and speaker at events around the world.

Through her work, Adriana has demonstrated a commitment to creating opportunities for women to succeed in business and life. Her passion for innovation, leadership, and women's empowerment has made her a respected figure in the business community, and her impact will undoubtedly continue to inspire and empower women for years to come.

Your Glow Is Unique

By Adriana Luna Carlos

When I think about the idea of a "healthy glow," I imagine something that radiates from within. It's not just about looking well-rested or having a perfect skincare routine; it's about the energy you carry, the confidence you exude, and the resilience that keeps you moving forward. For me, achieving a healthy glow has been a journey filled with challenges, self-discovery, and redefining what wellness truly means.

It's More Than Skin Deep

Wellness is often portrayed as an external achievement—a fit body, flawless skin, or a picture-perfect life. But what I've learned is that true wellness goes much deeper. It's about how you feel, not just how you look. It's about finding balance, peace, and strength in your life, even when things feel chaotic or uncertain.

For years, I struggled with my health in ways that weren't always visible to others. Heavy, prolonged periods that lasted months—at one point an entire year—drained me physically and emotionally. The fatigue, discomfort, and uncertainty left me feeling disconnected from my body. On top of that, dealing with infertility brought waves of sadness and disappointment. Having children was a dream I'd held onto for as long as I could remember, and facing the possibility that it might not happen was a heavy weight to carry.

It's experiences like these that taught me the importance of embracing wellness from the inside out. I realized that no matter how well I took care of my appearance, I couldn't truly glow if I wasn't taking care of my mind, body, and spirit.

The Power of Small Changes

When you're facing health challenges, it's easy to feel overwhelmed. There were times when I didn't know where to start or how to move forward. But I discovered that small, consistent changes can make a big difference. Wellness doesn't happen overnight—it's a journey of little steps that build over time.

For me, it started with acknowledging what my body needed and learning to listen to it. I began tracking my health patterns, noticing how different foods, activities, and stress levels affected how I felt. It wasn't about being perfect; it was about understanding what worked for me and making adjustments along the way.

One of the biggest shifts was learning to prioritize self-care. For years, I poured my energy into helping others, often neglecting my own needs. But I realized that to show up fully for the people I cared about, I had to take care of myself first. Self-care became non-negotiable—a daily practice that included simple things like drinking enough water, getting enough sleep, and setting boundaries.

Embracing Movement as Medicine

Exercise has always been a part of the conversation around wellness, but for me, it took on a new meaning. Instead of seeing movement as a way to achieve a certain body type, I began to view it as a way to care for my mental and physical health. Movement became medicine.

I started with gentle activities—things that felt good for my body rather than punishing it. Yoga helped me reconnect with myself, stretching out the tension I didn't realize I was holding. Walking outdoors became a way to clear my mind and soak in the healing power of nature. On days when I felt low energy, even five minutes of stretching made a difference.

Exercise wasn't just about improving my health—it became a tool for building confidence. Each time I showed up for myself, even when it was hard, I felt a little stronger. I learned that movement wasn't about perfection; it was about progress.

Healing Through Nourishment

Food has always been a big part of my life, but my relationship with it hasn't always been easy. Like many people, I've faced moments of emotional eating, stress-induced cravings, and the pressure to follow restrictive diets. But as I embarked on my wellness journey, I realized that food is more than fuel—it's a form of self-love.

I began focusing on nourishment rather than restriction. This wasn't about following a specific diet or eliminating entire food groups. It was about finding foods that made me feel good—energized, balanced, and satisfied. I experimented with new recipes, incorporated more whole foods, and allowed myself to enjoy treats without guilt.

The biggest lesson was learning to listen to my body. Cravings weren't something to fight against; they were signals. Was I dehydrated? Stressed? Lacking a certain nutrient? By paying attention to what my body was telling me, I was able to make choices that supported my overall well-being.

The Mental Battle: Overcoming Self-Doubt

While physical health was a big part of my journey, the mental battle was just as significant. Dealing with health challenges, infertility, and the pressures of daily life often left me feeling defeated. There were days when I doubted myself, when I felt like giving up, and when I questioned whether I'd ever truly feel "well."

What I've come to understand is that mental wellness is a practice. It's something you work on every day, and it's just as important as caring for your body. I started incorporating practices that helped me stay grounded, like journaling, meditation, and gratitude exercises. Writing down my thoughts became a way to process my emotions, and meditation helped me find moments of peace even on the hardest days.

I also leaned on affirmations—simple phrases that reminded me of my strength and worth. Saying things like "I am enough" or "I am resilient" might seem small, but over time, they rewired the way I thought about myself. They helped me shift from a place of self-doubt to one of self-compassion.

Confidence from Within

Confidence isn't something that comes from a new outfit, a number on a scale, or even a glowing complexion. True confidence comes from within—it's the result of embracing who you are, flaws and all. For me, confidence has been about showing up for myself every day, even when I don't feel like it. It's been about finding joy in the little things and celebrating progress rather than perfection.

There's something incredibly empowering about looking in the mirror and seeing not just your reflection, but your resilience. When I look at myself today, I see someone who has faced challenges and come out stronger. I see someone who is still growing, still learning, and still glowing from the inside out.

Practical Steps to Embrace Your Own Healthy Glow

If you're on a journey to wellness and confidence, know that it's okay to start small. Here are some practical steps that have helped me, and I hope they can help you too:

1. **Start with Self-Compassion:** Be kind to yourself. Acknowledge where you are without judgment and remind yourself that progress is more important than perfection.

2. **Create a Morning Routine:** Start your day with something that uplifts you, whether it's a few minutes of stretching, a

gratitude practice, or a healthy breakfast. Setting a positive tone for the day can make a big difference.

3. **Move in a Way That Feels Good:** Find activities that you enjoy and that energize you. Whether it's dancing, swimming, yoga, or walking, focus on how movement makes you feel rather than how it makes you look.

4. **Nourish Your Body:** Pay attention to how different foods make you feel. Choose meals that are satisfying and nourishing, and don't be afraid to enjoy treats in moderation.

5. **Prioritize Sleep:** Rest is essential for your body and mind. Create a bedtime routine that helps you wind down, and aim for 7-9 hours of sleep each night.

6. **Practice Gratitude:** Take a few moments each day to reflect on what you're grateful for. Gratitude can shift your perspective and help you focus on the positives in your life.

7. **Celebrate Small Wins:** Acknowledge every step forward, no matter how small. Each win is a reminder of your progress and your commitment to yourself.

8. **Set Boundaries:** Learn to say no to things that drain your energy and yes to things that align with your well-being.

9. **Surround Yourself with Positivity:** Spend time with people who uplift you and create an environment that supports your wellness journey.

10. **Stay Curious:** Wellness is a journey, not a destination. Stay open to learning, experimenting, and growing along the way.

Your journey to wellness and confidence is uniquely yours, and it's something to be celebrated. Remember that glowing from the inside out isn't about perfection—it's about embracing who you are, taking care of yourself, and finding joy in the process.

Every small step you take, every moment of self-care, brings you closer to the healthy glow you deserve. So be patient with yourself, honor your journey, and remember that your glow comes from the strength and beauty within you. Keep shining, because the world needs your light.

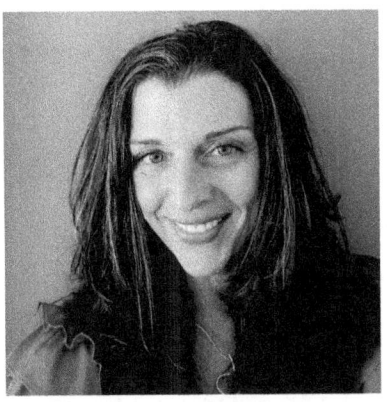

Kerry Martin

Founder of Wise Concierge Wellness LLC

https://www.linkedin.com/in/kerry-martin-rn-chc-28b8812a6/
https://www.facebook.com/profile.php?id=61553996403876
https://www.instagram.com/wiseconciergewellness/
https://wiseconciergewellness.com/

I am Kerry Martin, a Registered Nurse and Certified Health Coach, and the founder of Wise Concierge Wellness LLC, established in 2023. Frustrated by the gaps in our current healthcare system—particularly the absence of kindness and true self-care—I set out to create a practice that emphasizes holistic well-being.

My approach combines evidence-based clinical practices with mindfulness, tailoring sessions to meet my clients' unique needs. Whether you're navigating a stressful transition, feeling stuck in negative patterns, or seeking deeper self-understanding, I empower you to develop new skills and strategies that you can integrate into your daily life.

Together, we will identify the barriers holding you back, helping you connect with your inner self and discover the path that resonates with your heart.

Wellness Through Experience

By Kerry Martin

How my life used to be:

It's 5am and very cold here. I am awake because, like every day here, the bright fluorescent lights are switched on now. It is Thursday. I know that they are serving pancakes this morning, and it is one of the better meals. I also know it is cold and dark outside, and I am unsure if I want to eat or go back to sleep. I decide to brave the cold. After the cell doors are opened, I get in line to go to breakfast with the other women prisoners.

We are all here for different reasons, of course. We all made some seriously bad choices in our lives. Most of us have families and children we have left behind. The days here are gray and dark and long. There is some semblance of family and friendship if you want to get involved with other women in whatever capacity (friends, lovers, acquaintances). This can make the time go faster but also involves a level of drama I am unwilling to face. I have always been comfortable being alone, so I do my best to read, write, and exercise.

This was my life in a women's prison and as an alcoholic/drug addict. For years, I had abused alcohol and drugs. Over that time, I had some minor skirmishes with the law but I had up until now been able to avoid prison. Not this time. I was convicted and sentenced to 18 months. This is a story about my journey after leaving prison and how it is possible to accomplish what seems impossible.

How my life is now:

This morning I awoke at 6:30am in a room full of light. I have made the space around me inside and outside a haven. It is full of plants, water, sky, and nature in general. I surround myself with some artwork inside and out. After everyone leaves for work or school, the house is fairly quiet in the morning, except for my 3 dogs.

The first thing I do is get outside. I walk the dogs at a nearby trail or around the surrounding property. There are many animals here. Birds, deer, turkeys, chipmunks, squirrels, and the occasional bear. It is peaceful and serene. After our walk, I perform my daily ritual of meditation inside or outside, depending on the weather and how I am feeling. This is something that is non-negotiable. Without this and other important rituals on a daily basis, I become unmoored and not present in the moment. Then, I begin my workday.

How did I go from being incarcerated to living in a beautiful environment and doing the work I love? This is the story of how I found self-care and all that it means to me.

First, after leaving prison and some more struggling, I decided I was not going to use any substances anymore. I went to an outpatient program and followed every rule. I went to every meeting and sat through it all, even though I really did not want to be there. I had to be there if I wanted to change my life. Then, I got a decent job.

I got a dog, a labrador. That was such a valuable step. I had to be responsible for him. I had to get outside and walk him, feed him, and play with him. He was a great companion. He had to be walked no matter the weather and at least twice a day. Getting outside in nature is such an important part of my story.

I stopped spending time with negative people who were not on the same path as I was. I stopped going to places where I had gone when I used drugs or alcohol. I moved out of the town I had lived into a quiet place where I could be outside. I surrounded myself with beauty at my new home.

I started working out on a regular basis. I met people at the gym, and I also started being creative: writing, drawing, and making vision boards.

I made sure I ate whole, healthy foods, and drank a ton of water. I made sure I got 6–8 hours of sleep a night.

I apologized to friends and family for all the nonsense I put them through. I slowly gained their trust again. I worked very hard at this. It was not easy, but I am happy to say it was worth every emotional apology and clarification.

Things got better. I realized I wanted to go back to school and become a nurse after helping to care for my relative who was terminally ill. This new career was very meaningful to me. It resonated with me. I knew it was what I was meant to do. I knew the only way that this could happen was if I got a pardon.

I started the lengthy process of getting a pardon all on my own, without a lawyer. It was harder than getting into nursing school. Months of work, testimonials from friends and professionals, and extensive amounts of paperwork followed. Finally, the day came when I had to stand before a pardon board appointed by the governor. I was asked and answered many questions. I got the pardon!! It was absolutely one of the best days of my life.

Next was college/nursing school. I became an RN. Then, I worked at different hospital nursing positions. I kept taking different courses while I worked to become a Certified Health Coach. Courses in meditation and mindfulness. Cognitive Based Coaching. Positive Coaching.

Now I have my own business, Wise Concierge Wellness LLC. I help women with their health and wellness. It is the most rewarding thing I have ever done. I specialize in self-care for women. We work together and make individualized wellness plans. Some examples of my work: changing the way women think about putting themselves first, finding natural solutions for common health problems, making sure that women are making positive health decisions, and, where necessary, health changes.

In addition to my business, I plan to return to that prison soon to help the women there find health and wellness. Going through these life events was what has made me who I am. I hope this can help or inspire anyone who feels trapped or scared or thinks they can not get back on their feet. Anything is possible with time, positive guidance, and changes.

I embrace who I am and what I do! If you would like to improve your health and wellness and get tools to feel your best everyday contact:

kerry@wiseconciergewellness.com or
text/call confidential line 860-245-8525.

Website:
https://wiseconciergewellness.com/
Instagram:
www.instagram.com/wiseconciergewellness
Facebook:
https://www.facebook.com/profile.php?id=61553996403876&mibex
tid=LQQJ4d

Kerry lives in Connecticut with her amazing partner of 16 years and their 3 dogs.

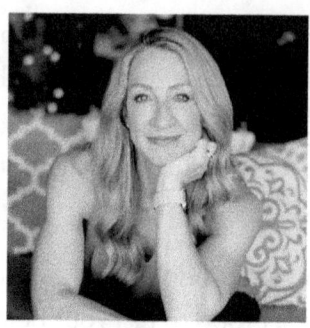

Jennifer Jenkins

Founder of Rooted Holistic Health Coaching

https://www.linkedin.com/in/jennifer-jenkins-rn-chc-fns-ryt-nlp-practitioner-1103825/
https://www.facebook.com/jejenkins1/
https://www.instagram.com/jen_jenkins_health_coach/
https://rootedholistichealth.com/

Jennifer Jenkins is a renowned leader in holistic wellness, dedicated to empowering individuals to reclaim their health and unlock their full potential. As a Registered Nurse, Health Coach, and Entrepreneur, Jennifer's mission is rooted in her own transformative healing journey, which led her to found Rooted Holistic Health Coaching. With over 25 years of experience, she specializes in addressing the root causes of metabolic imbalances, helping hundreds of clients break through limiting beliefs and restore optimal health.

Her unique approach goes beyond traditional methods, incorporating mindset shifts, nutrition, and holistic practices to achieve lasting results. Jennifer's programs are designed to address the body, mind, and spirit, providing a comprehensive solution to wellness.

As a sought-after speaker and workshop leader, she continues to inspire and guide others toward abundance and well-being in all aspects of life. Jennifer is committed to helping clients optimize their health and live vibrantly.

The Power Within: Reclaiming Your Health

By Jennifer Jenkins

Sometimes, it's in our darkest moments that the brightest lights begin to shine.

For five long years, I felt trapped—trapped in a cycle of illness, exhaustion, and frustration that seemed to have no end. Every day was a battle just to get through, and I constantly chased after answers, desperate for relief. In the process, I missed out on so many of life's beautiful moments. Holidays, milestones, and even the smallest, most joyful memories with my family slipped by while I was too sick, too tired, and too lost to truly live.

It felt like my body was betraying me. I had developed **Hashimoto's thyroiditis, leaky gut, food intolerances, severe allergies**, and **chronic sinusitis**. On top of that, I was battling **narcolepsy, depression, chronic fatigue, anemia, adrenal fatigue**, and **hormonal imbalances**. Every day, I felt weighed down by these health issues, and no matter how many doctors I saw or medications I tried, nothing seemed to improve. My life became a cycle of appointments, tests, and treatments, with no end in sight.

But as I reflect on those painful years now, I realize that there was more to the story. These physical conditions weren't just about the food I ate or the stress of everyday life. They were the result of something deeper that often gets overlooked: **years of significant trauma that I had carried within me**.

What we often fail to recognize is that trauma isn't just a mental or emotional wound—it manifests in the body. **Unresolved trauma can affect your nervous system, immune function, digestion, hormones, and energy levels**. The body remembers everything. While we may think we've "moved on" from painful experiences, our bodies are still holding onto the stress, fear, and pain, often silently—until it erupts into chronic illness or disease later in life.

At the time, I didn't realize that years of unresolved trauma had been quietly unraveling my health. Trauma doesn't just affect the mind; it manifests in the body in profound ways—through chronic inflammation, autoimmune conditions, digestive disorders, and hormonal imbalances. When trauma remains unresolved, the body stays locked in a **fight-or-flight** state, continuously releasing stress hormones that weaken the immune system and wreak havoc on your health. I had been operating in survival mode for so long, and my body was finally paying the price.

In those moments, it felt as though my health might never recover. But over the course of my career, I've come to understand that **there is no magic cure**. Despite what marketing might lead you to believe, healing doesn't come from a quick fix. It requires a deeper, more holistic approach.

As a Registered Nurse with over 25 years of experience, and through coaching hundreds of clients and completing advanced training in areas like neuroscience, HeartMath monitoring, nutrition, yoga, behavioral change, fitness, energy work, neuro-linguistic programming (NLP), and timeline therapy, I've learned one powerful truth: **True healing requires honoring the connection between the body, mind, and spirit**. It's not just about what we eat or how much we sleep. Healing is about addressing the whole person—physically, mentally, spiritually, and emotionally—and creating alignment between all aspects of our well-being.

After years of searching for answers, I realized that **my body could heal with the right lifestyle, and environmental, emotional, mental, and behavioral changes**. I discovered what I now call the "magic formula," but it wasn't a single solution or a one-size-fits-all approach. Healing required alignment—of my lifestyle, my thoughts, my environment—with what my body truly needed. That's why I always encourage people to discover what works best for them individually.

And, if you are working with a healthcare provider, it's crucial to consult with them before making any significant changes to ensure it complements your medical care.

Through this holistic lens, I found my way back to health, and now, it's my mission to share with you what I've learned. I've developed a simple blueprint of strategies you can start implementing today to improve your health and create lasting change. I call it **BREATHE.**

BREATHE: Your Blueprint for Health & Vitality

B – Breathe

Tuning into your breath is one of the most powerful tools for healing. When was the last time you truly paid attention to your breathing? Many of us unknowingly get stuck in shallow, unconscious breathing patterns that hold emotional energy and tension within our bodies. Significant emotional events, including trauma, often leave imprints on our breathing patterns, which can disrupt the balance of our nervous system. This dysregulation can create emotional blocks and, over time, contribute to the development of chronic diseases and various health issues.

By taking moments throughout the day to consciously pause and breathe deeply—filling your lungs fully and making your exhale longer than your inhale—can help you activate the parasympathetic nervous system. This simple yet powerful practice calms the nervous system, releases stored tension, and brings your body back into a state of relaxation and healing.

R – Reframe Your Mindset

Our mindset has the power to shape our reality. What we focus on expands. If your thoughts constantly revolve around negativity, illness, or limiting beliefs, these patterns will continue to dominate your life.

One of the most powerful ways to shift your mindset is by **reframing negative thoughts** into empowering ones. The next time a negative thought arises, ask yourself, "How can I view this differently and transform it into an empowering statement?"

For example, a common statement I hear from clients when they first come to me is, "I can't...lose weight, sleep, manage my stress, etc." When we say things like "I can't" or "I am" in a limiting way, we are essentially convincing ourselves that these statements are true. That's why it's essential to become mindful of our thoughts and recognize how they shape our reality.

In your health and wellness journey, learning to replace self-doubt and fear with thoughts of **possibility, hope, and empowerment** is critical. **Your thoughts either fuel your healing or keep you stuck**—the choice is yours.

E – Environment Matters

Who we surround ourselves with has a profound impact on our health and well-being. Take a moment to reflect on the people you spend the most time with. Are they uplifting and supportive, or do they drain your energy? Are they aligned with your health goals, or are they influencing habits that don't serve your well-being? The people in your life shape your mindset, behaviors, and overall environment—so it's crucial to be intentional about the energy you allow into your space.

Your environment can either support or hinder your growth. If you surround yourself with people who inspire you, encourage healthy habits, and share a positive outlook, it becomes easier to stay motivated and make lasting changes. On the other hand, if you are surrounded by negativity, resistance, or unhealthy influences, it can be challenging to stay on track, no matter how dedicated you are.

One powerful way to shift your environment is to **seek out like-minded individuals who are on a similar health journey**. This could mean joining a local fitness group, a meditation class, or a nutrition-focused meet-up. Surrounding yourself with people who share similar goals creates a sense of accountability and community, which can be invaluable when you face challenges along the way. You may also consider finding **online support groups**—there are countless forums, communities, and programs dedicated to health, wellness, and personal growth. These spaces allow you to connect with others from around the world who are striving toward similar goals, providing support, advice, and encouragement.

Another aspect of environment is creating physical spaces that promote health. For example, organizing your home in a way that encourages healthy behaviors—like having fresh, nutritious food easily accessible or setting up a dedicated space for yoga, meditation, or exercise—can make a big difference in your ability to maintain healthy habits.

Remember, **you become like the people and energy you surround yourself with**. If you want to make positive changes in your life, it's important to surround yourself with people and environments that uplift, support, and inspire you. Whether it's joining a group with shared values, cultivating friendships with those who motivate you, or creating physical spaces that encourage healthy habits, your environment plays a critical role in your success. Be intentional about who and what you allow into your life, and watch how much easier it becomes to stay aligned with your health goals.

A – Always Stay Hydrated

One of the most important things you can do for your health is to **make hydration a daily priority**. Drinking **purified water** is especially important, as it is free from harmful chemicals, toxins, and pollutants that can be present in tap water. Purified water helps your body stay clean and balanced, ensuring that your systems are not burdened with unnecessary contaminants. Clean water plays a crucial role in helping your kidneys and liver detoxify your body, and it allows your cells to maintain balance and perform optimally.

Aim to drink at least half your body weight in ounces of water daily (unless otherwise indicated by your healthcare provider). For example, if you weigh 150 pounds, you should aim to drink around 75 ounces of water each day. This ensures that your body has the fluid it needs to support vital functions like:

- **Digestion**: Water aids in breaking down food so that your body can absorb nutrients more effectively. Without enough water, digestion can slow down, leading to bloating, constipation, or discomfort.

- **Metabolism**: Hydration plays a key role in your metabolism, the process through which your body converts food into energy. Staying properly hydrated helps your metabolism work efficiently, which can support weight management and overall energy levels.

- **Detoxification**: Your body's natural detox pathways rely on water to flush out toxins and waste products. By drinking enough purified water, you support your liver and kidneys in cleansing your body, which is vital for long-term health.

- **Energy Levels**: Even mild dehydration can lead to fatigue and low energy levels. Water is essential for maintaining optimal brain function and overall energy, keeping you alert and focused throughout the day.

- **Cellular Function**: Every cell in your body depends on water to perform its specific roles. Water is the foundation of cellular health—it helps transport nutrients into cells and waste products out, allowing each cell to operate efficiently and stay healthy.

Staying properly hydrated also **supports your skin**, as water is essential for maintaining elasticity and hydration, which can reduce the appearance of fine lines and promote a radiant complexion. Hydration helps lubricate your joints and supports muscle function, making it crucial for physical activity and recovery.

In addition to drinking purified water, it's important to note that hydration also comes from foods like fruits and vegetables, which are naturally high in water content and nutrients that support hydration.

Making sure you stay hydrated isn't just about avoiding thirst—it's about giving your body the foundational element it needs to function properly, cleanse itself, and maintain energy. **Start today by making hydration a non-negotiable part of your routine**, and your body will thank you for it.

T – Take Time for Movement

Movement is truly medicine for the body, mind, and spirit. It goes far beyond just "working out"—movement is essential for maintaining your overall health, vitality, and longevity. Aim to move your body for at least 30 minutes each day, whether through walking, yoga, dancing, strength training, or any activity that gets your body in motion. Even better, take your movement outdoors and connect with nature while you move, as nature provides grounding energy that helps calm the nervous system and supports mental clarity.

One of the most important aspects of movement is **functional movement**—the kind of movement that mirrors natural, everyday activities and strengthens your body in a way that enhances your ability to perform daily tasks. Functional movements, such as squatting, lifting, pulling, and pushing, help improve balance, coordination, and strength, which are critical for maintaining **mobility** and **independence** as we age. This type of movement helps protect your joints and muscles from injury and deterioration, promoting longevity and quality of life.

Connecting with nature while you move amplifies these benefits. The fresh air, sunlight, and grounding energy of the natural environment provide additional mental and physical health benefits. **Nature calms the nervous system**, helping to reduce stress levels and foster a sense of peace and clarity.

Ultimately, **movement is a cornerstone of long-term health and well-being**. By integrating functional movement into your daily routine—whether it's through a brisk walk, a yoga session, or a strength workout—you are setting yourself up for a healthier, more vibrant life. Prioritizing movement not only keeps your body strong and resilient, but it also nurtures your mind and spirit, empowering you to feel more connected to yourself and the world around you.

H – Have a Meditation Practice

Meditation isn't just about relaxation—it's a tool for **deep personal growth** and well-being. When practiced consistently, meditation promotes **neuroplasticity**, meaning it helps your brain form new neural pathways. This enhances your brain's capacity to adapt, learn, and build resilience in the face of stress or adversity. Over time, meditation can literally reshape your brain, increasing the gray matter in areas associated with emotional regulation, self-awareness, and empathy.

Additionally, meditation helps **enhance emotional resilience** by allowing you to observe your thoughts and feelings without judgment. This non-reactive awareness reduces the emotional reactivity that often triggers stress and anxiety, enabling you to respond to challenges more calmly and thoughtfully. It also provides space to acknowledge difficult emotions, such as fear or anger, and release them in a healthy, constructive way.

Meditation has also been shown to support **physical health** by lowering blood pressure, improving sleep quality, and even boosting the immune system. When you meditate, you activate the **parasympathetic nervous**

system, which helps your body enter a state of rest and repair. This is where healing occurs on a deep cellular level, allowing your body to recover from stress and function more efficiently.

Incorporating meditation into your daily routine, even for just a few minutes, can have ripple effects on every aspect of your life. It supports not only **mental and emotional well-being** but also physical health, offering a holistic approach to healing and transformation. Whether you are looking to manage stress, improve focus, or cultivate deeper emotional awareness, meditation is a practice that offers lasting benefits for your body, mind, and spirit.

E – Eat Clean and Sleep Well

Nutrition and sleep are the foundation of good health, forming the building blocks for how well your body functions, heals, and regenerates. When it comes to nutrition, focus on eating clean, whole foods that come from the earth—think **organic, minimally processed proteins**, healthy fats, and a variety of colorful vegetables with each meal. These nutrient-dense foods provide your body with the essential vitamins, minerals, and antioxidants needed to support energy, immune function, and overall vitality.

To optimize your nutrition, aim to **minimize highly processed foods**, refined sugars, and artificial additives that can lead to inflammation, blood sugar imbalances, and poor digestion. Prioritize quality over quantity, making sure your meals are balanced with protein, healthy fats, and fiber-rich vegetables, which help stabilize your blood sugar throughout the day. Additionally, consider incorporating fermented foods like sauerkraut or kefir to support gut health, as a healthy gut plays a critical role in overall well-being and immune function.

One key tip to improve both your digestion and sleep quality is to **avoid eating within 2–3 hours of bedtime**. This gives your body time to properly digest your last meal, preventing discomfort, acid reflux, or indigestion that can disrupt your sleep. Proper digestion also supports better nutrient absorption, leaving you feeling more energized and less sluggish the next day.

Sleep is equally vital to your health. Aim for 7–8 hours of restful sleep each night, as this is when your body does its most powerful healing and repair work. During sleep, your brain processes information, your muscles recover, and your immune system strengthens, allowing you to wake up feeling refreshed and rejuvenated. A well-rested body is better equipped to handle stress, maintain balanced hormones, and support overall well-being.

To improve your sleep quality, consider the following tips:

- **Create a bedtime routine**: Developing a consistent evening routine signals to your body that it's time to wind down. This could include relaxing activities like reading, meditating, or practicing gentle yoga. Avoid screens (phones, TVs, or computers) at least an hour before bed, as blue light can interfere with your body's production of melatonin, the sleep hormone.

- **Make your sleep environment calming**: Your bedroom should be a space of rest and relaxation. Keep the room cool, dark, and quiet, and invest in a comfortable mattress and pillows. Consider using a white noise machine or a sleep mask if external noises or light are disruptive.

- **Limit caffeine and alcohol**: Caffeine can linger in your system for hours, so it's best to avoid it in the afternoon and evening. Alcohol might make you feel sleepy initially, but it can disrupt your sleep cycles and lead to poor-quality rest. Instead, opt for herbal teas or water in the evening.

- **Practice stress management**: High levels of stress and anxiety can make it difficult to fall asleep or stay asleep. Incorporating relaxation techniques like deep breathing, meditation, or journaling into your nightly routine can help calm your mind and prepare your body for restful sleep.

By prioritizing **clean, nutrient-dense foods** and establishing a **healthy sleep routine**, you set the stage for your body to function optimally, heal more effectively, and feel more resilient in the face of daily stress. Both nutrition and sleep are essential pillars of long-term health and well-being, and small improvements in these areas can lead to profound changes in your energy levels, mental clarity, and overall vitality.

This **BREATHE** blueprint is simple, but it addresses the most important areas of your life that contribute to your overall well-being. When you take a holistic approach—incorporating breath, mindset, environment, hydration, movement, meditation, sleep, and nutrition—you empower your body to heal itself from the inside out. Healing isn't about perfection or doing everything at once. It's about making small, consistent changes that align your lifestyle with your body's natural rhythms and needs.

You are more powerful than you think, and with these tools, you can start improving your health today. **BREATHE**—and begin your journey to healing and vitality.

As I look back on my journey, one thing stands out above all else: **our health is the greatest investment we will ever make**. It's the foundation of everything—our happiness, our relationships, our ability to live life fully and with purpose. Without our health, even the most precious moments can lose their spark, and the dreams we hold dear feel just out of reach.

But here's the empowering truth: **You hold the power to change your health, and in doing so, change your life**. Healing doesn't have to be overwhelming, and it certainly doesn't happen overnight. It's the small, consistent changes you make every single day that lead to big transformations over time. Each decision—whether it's taking a few deep breaths to calm your mind, choosing nutrient-dense foods, drinking more water, or prioritizing rest—brings you closer to the vibrant health and life you deserve.

So, I encourage you to start now. **Don't wait for the perfect moment or the perfect plan.** Just start where you are. Commit to making small, mindful changes that honor your body, mind, and spirit. Whether it's a 10-minute walk outside, reframing a negative thought, or setting aside time to meditate, each step you take matters.

Remember, **you are worth it**. Your health is worth it. Every bit of energy you put into caring for yourself will pay dividends—not just in how you feel physically but also in your emotional well-being, resilience, and joy for life.

You don't have to have all the answers right now. You just need to take that first step. And then another. And before you know it, those small changes will add up to something extraordinary.

The journey to reclaiming your health is the most rewarding journey you'll ever take. You are capable, you are strong, and you are worthy of living a life full of vitality and purpose. **Invest in yourself today**—one step, one breath, one choice at a time—and watch as your life transforms in ways you never thought possible.

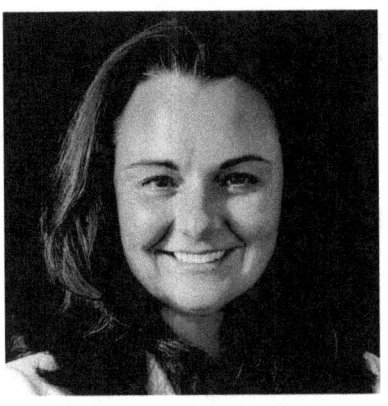

Natalie Horseman

Mentor & Founder of Hollowed Horseman Publishing
MSN, RN, CNOR, Coach

https://www.instagram.com/theselfdoubtdetox
https://horsemanbooks.com/

Natalie Horseman, MSN, RN, CNOR is a dedicated nurse with nearly two decades of experience in child and family development. Her extensive background in healthcare has equipped her with a profound understanding of resilience and strength. Throughout her career, Natalie has been committed to guiding individuals through life's most challenging moments with both compassion and empathy. Her personal journey of overcoming adversity has deeply fueled her passion for empowering others. Through her writing, Natalie combines practical advice with heartfelt encouragement, creating a sense of community for those navigating life's storms. She believes that while our experiences shape us, they do not define us. Through her contributions, Natalie strives to inspire readers to embrace their inner strength and resilience, offering reassurance that they are never alone on their journey.

The Silent Unraveling

By Natalie Horseman

Echoes of Ambition

Independence, education, and self-sufficiency were ingrained in me from an early age. These were non-negotiable values, a blueprint for life. Dedication to one's career wasn't just an expectation—it was the ultimate measure of success. When I chose nursing, a profession that blended compassion with challenge, I believed I had found my calling. Yet, as I embarked on my journey, I discovered that the path would push me to my limits in ways I could have never anticipated.

My first job as a pediatric nurse was a whirlwind—a blur of tiny humans, anxious parents, and organized chaos. It was exhilarating, terrifying, and utterly addictive. The long hours and demanding shifts quickly became the norm, but the satisfaction of a job well done kept me going. I volunteered for weekends, holidays, and the toughest shifts, sacrificing my personal life so my colleagues could be with their families. Looking back, it's ironic: Though I had no children of my own, I prioritized the well-being of those who did.

After graduate school, I eagerly stepped into a leadership position. I packed up my life and my dog, relocating to a new state with excitement and determination. This was a crucial career step, and I was committed to climbing the professional ladder, no matter the cost.

The Cost of Dedication

When I say I gave my life to that job, I mean it quite literally. I was there before sunrise and often left long after sunset. Days blurred into a haze of emergencies, meetings, and never-ending tasks. The department's needs, the well-being of the children, and the demands of the physicians all felt like personal emergencies, and I took it upon myself to fix everything.

My dedication became a badge of honor. I took pride in being available 24/7—the ultimate problem-solver and "Yes Woman". But, beneath the surface, a storm was brewing. The emotional toll slowly crept in, manifesting as chronic fatigue and anxiety. The spark in my eyes dimmed under the weight of relentless responsibility.

As the pressure mounted, I withdrew from friends and family, convinced I could handle everything alone. My life became a relentless routine, each day indistinguishable from the last. My job consumed me, becoming my entire identity. On the outside, I appeared to be a successful professional. But inside, I was on the brink of collapse, hiding the cracks in my foundation behind a polished exterior.

The Wake-Up Call

The turning point came during a lecture on physician well-being. As the department head listed the signs of burnout, it felt like a slap across the face. Every symptom she described resonated deeply with me—the exhaustion, the cynicism, the constant feeling of being on edge. I had heard the term "burnout" before, but I had never grasped its full impact on mental, physical, and emotional health until that moment.

Conversations with my mentors were another wake-up call. They saw the exhaustion etched on my face, the smile that had vanished, replaced by a weariness that clung to me. Their genuine concern reflected back the truth I had been avoiding: I was losing not just my passion, but my very sense of self.

Therapy became my sanctuary, a place to process the emotional overload and the toll my career had taken. My therapist helped me understand the importance of setting boundaries and prioritizing my own well-being. For years, I had been so focused on taking care of everyone else that I had completely neglected myself.

Taking a step back was the hardest decision I had ever made, but also the most liberating. For years, I had defined myself by my career, allowing it to dictate where I lived, how I spent my time, and even who I was. But when I moved again—this time for myself and not for my job—it marked the beginning of a profound transformation.

With a more manageable schedule, I finally had the space to breathe, to rediscover who I was beyond the confines of a job title. Those first few months were an emotional rollercoaster. Guilt gnawed at me—guilt for not pushing harder, for leaving the office before the sun set, for not being 'enough' in the way I had always measured success. But as the weeks passed, I began to shed the layers of my old identity. Slowly, almost imperceptibly at first, I started to reclaim my life.

The Unselfish Journey

This journey toward well-being is a constant work in progress. There are still days when old habits creep back in, and the temptation to overextend myself is strong. But with each sunrise, I make a conscious choice to prioritize my mental and emotional health, to choose my own happiness.

Burnout is insidious, a silent thief that steals your joy, energy, and sense of self. But it doesn't have to be the end of the story. By making your well-being a top priority, you can reclaim your sparkle and rediscover a life filled with joy and purpose. Remember, you are not defined by your job title or achievements; you are a whole person, deserving of balance and happiness.

Self-care isn't selfish; it's essential. Prioritizing your whole self creates a positive ripple effect in your life. Looking back, I realize that my drive for perfection and the constant need to prove myself were my biggest obstacles. In striving to be the best nurse and leader, I lost touch with my own identity. It took years to rediscover who I was outside of my career.

To anyone feeling overwhelmed, overworked, and underappreciated: It's okay to not be okay. It's okay to say no and to take time for yourself. Don't wait until you're at the breaking point like I did.

You're not a superhero; you're a human being with needs and limitations, and that's perfectly alright. Let's redefine success not by how much we achieve, but by how much joy we experience along the way. So, take a deep breath, treat yourself with grace, and give yourself permission to rest. You deserve it.

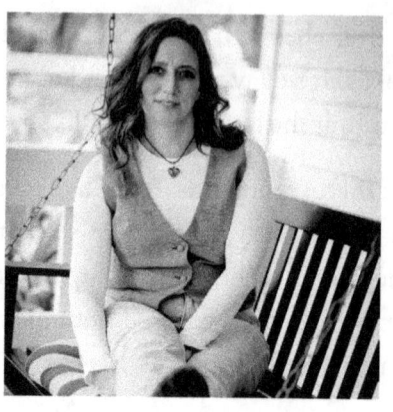

Kimberly Beam

KimBeam.com
Intuition and Mediation Coach

https://www.linkedin.com/in/kimberly-beam-5575144/
https://www.facebook.com/iamkimbeam
https://www.instagram.com/iamkimbeam
https://www.kimbeam.com/

Kim Beam is on a spiritual journey in this lifetime that is opening the doors of her heart and spirit to all of life's supportive experiences. She holds 2 masters degrees - one in creative writing and one in social work. She is a Hodgkin's Lymphoma survivor. Kim offers the world her gifts by being a public speaker, an intuitive reader, a reiki master, a healer, and an adventurer of the spiritual realms through meditation, teachings, trainings, and being grounded in her body. She is a manifestor and believes in abundance for everyone.

Creating Your Healthy Glow from Within: From Anxiety to Peace

By Kimberly Beam

In May of 2010, when I was 33, I was diagnosed with Hodgkin's Lymphoma. I went through treatment, survived, and came out the other side—but I was not the same person who came out of treatment as the person who went in.

Long before treatment, I was anxious. I had an undiagnosed anxiety disorder my whole life. It was only really acknowledged in my early twenties. At that time, not only was I swallowed by panic attacks, but I also created cycles of panic, fearing when the next one would come. Medication management was the only strategy the doctors offered, and I would go on and off the meds regularly.

There was a moment after the chemo for Hodgkin's was over when I was standing in the oncologist's office, and I turned to Dr. N and said, "I think I have post-traumatic stress."

My mom said, "We're actually calling it Post Traumatic Cancer Disorder."

My oncologist pressed her lips together in sympathy and nodded her head in agreement. She asked what I was doing for the baseline anxiety.

I named the SSRI (selective serotonin reuptake inhibitor) I had been prescribed.

Then she said, "What are you doing for the breakthrough anxiety?"

I looked at her, shocked, "You know about that?"

She said, "I'm a hematologist oncologist."

The only answer I had at that time to, "What are you doing about your anxiety?" was medication management. But let me be honest, SSRIs and

Benzodiazepines and I do not get along. The side effects and long-term effects wreak havoc on my overall mental health.

It wasn't until I got into studying for my master's in Social Work that I got to know what post-traumatic stress actually is. What I learned was the moment you think, "I could die," in any given situation, that's the moment that post-traumatic stress has the potential to grab hold. There are a number of other factors that determine if a person develops PTS symptoms, like coping strategies and resilience, but if there's the thought, "I could die," the door for PTS symptoms opens. (I don't put the D on PTSD, which stands for Disorder. I do not call it a "disorder." It's a normal reaction to abnormal circumstances.)

After discovering all of this, I wanted my body to learn how to manage the memories and the emotions.

One of the ways I've always coped with overwhelm is by writing—it helps move the emotions out of my body. I wrote the trauma narrative, and it became a book— *What the Doctors Don't Tell You: One Woman's Journey Through the Hodgkin's Lymphoma.*

That wasn't enough. I was still struggling with panic and anxiety.

One of the life changes I made because of being diagnosed and treated for Hodgkin's was I left being an English teacher and enrolled in a master's program in Social Work. One night in my Child Welfare class, the professor brought in a trauma-informed yoga instructor, and she led us through some exercises to be present in our bodies. She led us through some alternate nostril breathing, other deep breathing techniques, and basic yoga poses like Tree and Mountain. She also guided us through some mindfulness-based stress reduction activities—basically meditation in a scientifically researched package.

What I learned from just this 30-minute exercise was the power of my breath to break my anxiety cycles. I also learned the power of allowing my body to be what it is—to not put pressure on it, to not put expectations on it, to just let it be what it is.

People I have shared these practices with have agreed that they give relief.

Because of these experiences, I decided to become a mindfulness instructor and am now a qualified MBSR instructor through UMass Medical School. I've gone on two seven-day silent retreats and made my own five-week mostly silent retreat. (I talked about an hour a day on the five-week retreat.) I also have a daily meditation practice where I sit for at least 30 minutes most days, and I try to practice for a consecutive hour on the weekends.

All of this meditation practice has taught me my brain never shuts up. It wants to analyze everything. It also catastrophizes and makes up worst-case scenarios that increase my anxiety. I have come to learn that my brain is a big, fat liar—it just lets me down all the time. It also insults me and is cruel. It makes up stories that make me feel terrible and I believe them, just because it's my brain saying them.

Russ Harris, in his book, *The Illustrated Happiness Trap*, says that if you take your brain out of your body, put it in somebody else's body, and then have your brain speak out of that person's mouth—we wouldn't be friends with that person.

However, because we're talking about the thoughts in our own heads, we believe them.

Every time.

My consistent meditation practice also has made it possible for me to come off all anxiety medications.

Don't get me wrong, the panic still sometimes comes in.

I feel it better. I manage it better. I see my stress levels and work on them when they are small. But, I still occasionally have a panic attack. But instead of being sucked under by them, I have learned how to break their cycles.

It comes down to breathwork and dedication to taking time to practice.

When we breathe using our lower bellies, we increase oxygen all over our bodies, and we decrease the amount of carbon dioxide in our bodies. When we breathe in our upper chest (which is a part of the fear response: freeze, flight, and fight), we increase the carbon dioxide and decrease the amount of oxygen in our bodies. High CO2 triggers the stress response, which in turn creates anxiety, panic, and decreases oxygen throughout the whole body. Opposite to that, high oxygen levels increase the relaxation response. The more oxygen in your body, the more you are telling your body you are safe. So, deep belly breaths (which feel unnatural at first) increase your oxygen levels and break the panic cycle.

My work with meditation and breath work has created a different landscape both inside and outside my body. It has allowed me to shine internal peace. Dear reader, that is my wish for you. So many people are not able to create their own inner calm. By listening in meditation and to my intuition, I have been able to walk in my true purpose. My life vision is to help others see the path to their true purpose and happiness. I give intuitive readings and offer additional services to help individuals find their peace, contentment, and, ultimately, their Healthy Glow. If you visit KimBeam.com, you will find at the top of the homepage a free guide to bring more peace into your life.

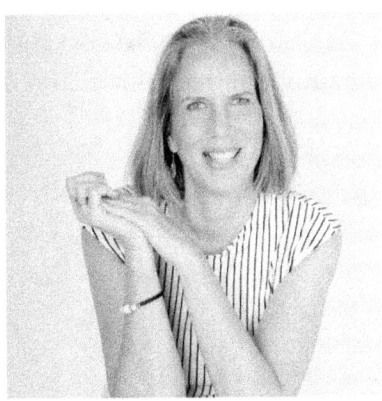

Astrid Boot

Astrid Boot
Spiritual Healer & Teacher

https://au.linkedin.com/in/astrid-boot-06370bb7
https://www.facebook.com/AstridBootHealer
https://www.instagram.com/astridboot9/
https://astridboot.com.au
https://astridboot.com.au/her-healthy-glow/

Astrid Boot is a spiritual healer & teacher who has had her own practice since 2006 in the Netherlands and from 2011 in Wollongong, NSW, Australia.

Astrid facilitates empathetic adults and children who've had a traumatic experience, to heal and to let go of the pain, so they stand in their power again and feel at peace.

She doesn't want to give up until her clients have reached their goals and she provides useful exercises and spiritual wisdom during her sessions. She believes setting intentions for the outcome of her clients' sessions is powerful and she expects miracles to happen.

Being a part of the complete transformation process with the end result of a happy and confident client, brings Astrid fulfillment.

Besides sessions with clients, Astrid also teaches courses and workshops. Furthermore, she is the author of the children's book 'Meghan's Miracle Week'.

Astrid works in person and online internationally.

How to Personally Grow to Glow

By Astrid Boot

Relationships Are Opportunities for Personal Growth

Growing up in a small farming village where the belief was to stay married for the rest of your life with the same person, turned out to be not my truth and reality. It was a challenging path because I had no one in my circles who could help with dealing with breakups, and there was a lot of gossip in the village. At times, I suffered from intense emotions like distrust, sadness, fear, and low self-esteem. My confidence had left the building. Several times in my life, I've climbed up the ladder of self-esteem and increased my confidence. Nine years after my husband passed away, I can say I've dealt with many emotions, chronic health issues, blocking beliefs, and disconnection from my spiritual side. I have my spark back, increased my confidence to a level higher than ever before, and I get the feedback that I am radiant.

What Do You Do with Emotions in Relationships?

It has been a journey of learning through relationships. You might have discovered in life that you learn through relationships with partners, family, your children, friends, and others. In every romantic relationship, you start at a level where you resonate with each other. You fall in love, feel amazing, glow, and experience a boost in your energy.

Then during your relationship, you start to know each other more, and the differences between you come up. Emotions come to the surface, and now it is about communication between the two of you. I don't know about you, but I definitely hadn't learned from my parents how to express my emotions. I had seen how they didn't speak to each other for days when there was a disagreement, and how they avoided each other in the same house.

What happens in your body when you experience an emotion? You notice a feeling in a part of your body. It asks your attention, but do you listen and act upon it? My advice is to say what you feel, a simple "I feel angry right now," or "I feel so overwhelmed now," gives your emotion some relief and a way out.

If you keep emotions inside, they will get triggered in a future situation and grow bigger inside. If this keeps happening, there comes a time when the emotion gets triggered and explodes. Think about someone exploding with anger in a situation where that feeling is out of place.

From my own experience I've learned that emotions caused intolerances in my physical body for certain foods, which resulted in deficiencies of vitamins and minerals. After releasing the emotions connected to those intolerances, my physical body could absorb the nutrients from food again and restore the levels of vitamins and minerals to the right amounts.

The Self-Help Tools That Work Best for Me

I am a fan of simple and efficient methods when it comes to self-help tools. When I discovered EFT Tapping, I started using it for situations in my life where I had emotions or thoughts, or both. How I use it, is sitting quietly and starting to tap on the acupressure points used with EFT Tapping, while focusing on what I feel in my body and what thoughts come up. When I start, I measure the intensity on a scale from 0-100. I keep tapping till it feels neutral, and on a scale from 0-100, I've reached the zero point. It's not always possible to reach this zero point in one tapping session, so you just continue another time later that day and other days till you feel neutral and have reached the desired zero point. Especially with tapping on losses, fears, financial struggles, distrust, disconnection from my spiritual side, and lack of confidence, I've achieved breakthroughs to happiness, love, internal peace, and more flow about finances, trust, faith, connection with my spiritual side, and a huge increase of confidence.

Another self-help tool that I'm very grateful for is Reiki. On a daily basis, I use Reiki on myself. It helps to relax, get a quieter mind, and ground well so it feels I'm connected strongly with the earth. I teach Reiki at all levels and would love to see every child would learn this as a self-help tool.

If you're in a state of intense emotions, you often feel weak inside. After losing my husband, people in my circles said that I was so strong, but I felt the opposite. It was years later and a lot of working on releasing emotions and blocking beliefs, that I could see my own strength. I've always stayed optimistic; when I felt miserable, I thought, 'Next week, I'll feel better, it's only temporary.' What also helped was staying in a daily routine: getting up even though I had been awake for hours, and making breakfast for my daughter, helping her to go to school. Going on a walk along the beach and just sitting there, staring at the water, and sending everything that was bothering me into the water, was helpful too.

Getting My Spark Back by the Creativity That Brings Joy

A year after my husband passed, I asked myself how I could get my spark back and what would bring me joy. I realised I missed singing and dancing, and I arranged private lessons for both. It is important to do something creative to have your creativity flow again, whether it's colouring in, painting, drawing, sewing, dancing, music, or something else.

You have the power to get through everything and come out at the other side more empowered, more confident, and with a higher frequency. Take the time to work on yourself every day. Sit quietly with your feelings and thoughts and release them, let them go. Check in with your own spiritual connection where you want to receive guidance from, because we all have guidance available. As the last piece of advice: Ask for help from your guides and people around you. Believe in yourself to have everything in you to shine!

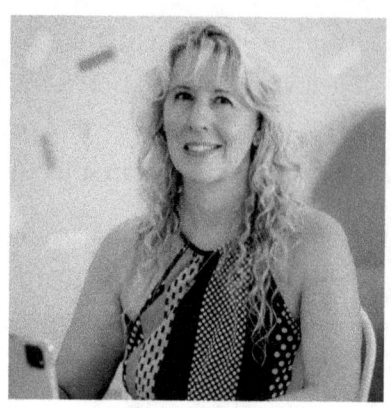

Erica Elliott

WarriorHeart Healing Hearts, LLC
Owner & Coach

https://www.linkedin.com/in/erica-elliott-ms-lpc-b90911150
https://www.facebook.com/warriorheartxo
https://www.instagram.com/warriorheartxo
https://warriorheart-ignite.passion.io/
https://linktr.ee/WarriorHeartxo

I have a Masters in Counseling Psychology, Licensed Counselor, Certified Brain Health Coach and Certified Alternative Medicines Professional trained in a plethora of modalities, other certifications. I take a very wholistic approach to mind, body, and spirit helping people heal. With over 30 years of experience working with thousands of people over the years, this has never been a job for me but a Calling, because I absolutely am overjoyed to help people grow, heal soar and live the most amazing life God has always intended them to have! I myself have overcome lots of trials, traumas and triggers and know healing takes place as we have a compassionate relationship with another to guide us and help us strengthen ourselves to wholeness and vitality. Like iron sharpening iron we create a healing that changes our legacy and the legacy of those around us.

How to W.I.N. at Self-Care Every Day: Transform Your Life with Simple Daily Routines

By Erica Elliott

Do you ever feel like you're constantly trying to do everything, pushing yourself to the limit, only to end up exhausted, overwhelmed, and frustrated? You're not alone. Many people find themselves in this cycle, struggling to juggle the demands of life with the need for personal well-being. As a counselor with over 30 years of experience, I've worked with thousands of people who face these same challenges. I, too, have experienced the toll of this relentless pace, especially after a life-altering experience following a bout with COVID-19 in 2020. I want to share my journey and offer practical strategies for incorporating self-care into your daily routine, so you can live a more balanced, energized, and fulfilling life.

For much of my life, self-care was a concept I preached but didn't fully practice. I was high-energy, driven by an ADHD-fueled need to stay busy, and influenced by a "suck it up and drive on" mentality ingrained during my time in the military. Self-care seemed like a luxury, something I could attend to when there was time, which, of course, there never was. But when COVID-19 hit, everything changed. The virus left me with a host of long-term symptoms, including adrenal fatigue, hyperkalemia, hypothyroidism, tinnitus, chronic migraines, and debilitating fatigue. I was forced to confront the reality that my body and mind could no longer sustain the relentless pace I had set for myself. My old strategies of pushing through and ignoring my body's signals no longer worked—in fact, they made things worse.

The more I tried to push myself, the more my body resisted, like a stubborn mule refusing to budge. I had to learn the hard way that self-care wasn't optional; it was essential if I wanted to regain my health and live a better quality of life. This realization was a turning point for me, both personally and professionally. It deepened my understanding of the importance of self-care, not just as a concept, but as a daily practice that can make the difference between thriving and merely surviving.

The Importance of Self-Care

Research on burnout has become increasingly important in recent years, revealing its significant impact on health both globally and within the United States. Burnout is characterized by emotional exhaustion, cynicism, and a sense of reduced efficacy. It affects a substantial portion of the workforce, with studies showing that more than half of employees in various sectors experience its symptoms. Globally, burnout has been linked to a range of health problems, including anxiety, depression, and cardiovascular issues. In the United States, the rise of remote work and increased job demands during the COVID-19 pandemic have exacerbated these challenges, leading organizations to rethink workplace practices. The growing awareness of burnout's consequences has sparked greater advocacy for mental health resources, work-life balance initiatives, and supportive workplace cultures aimed at fostering well-being and productivity.

Despite this increased focus on burnout and self-care, many people still struggle to incorporate self-care into their daily lives. This is often because they view self-care as something time-consuming or extravagant, like a spa day or a weekly massage. While these activities are certainly beneficial, they're not practical for most people on a daily basis. True self-care is about the small, consistent actions you take every day to nurture your mind, body, and spirit. It's about creating habits that support your overall well-being, so you can show up as your best self in all areas of your life.

Introducing W.I.N.: A Simple Self-Care Framework

To help myself and others build a life centered around consistent self-care, I developed a simple framework using the acronym W.I.N., which stands for Welcome, Intention, and Nighttime rituals. This framework is designed to be easy to remember and implement, allowing you to incorporate self-care into your daily routine without feeling overwhelmed.

Welcome: Starting Your Day with Self-Care

The first step in the W.I.N. framework is to Welcome the day. This means beginning each morning with a mindset of positivity and gratitude. Before you even get out of bed, take a moment to welcome the day with enthusiasm. Tell yourself, "This is going to be a great day," or recite a mantra like, "This is the day that the Lord has made; I will rejoice and be glad in it." By starting your day with a positive mindset, you set the tone for how the rest of your day will unfold.

Visualization is another powerful tool you can use in the morning. As you lie in bed, take a few minutes to visualize your day going smoothly. See yourself moving through your tasks with energy and ease, enjoying your interactions with others, and taking breaks when needed. Visualize yourself feeling balanced and fulfilled at the end of the day. This simple practice can help you approach your day with a sense of calm and purpose rather than feeling rushed or stressed.

Prayer can also be an important part of your morning self-care routine. Welcoming God or a higher power to guide your day with ease can provide a sense of peace and direction. Over the years, I've found that when I start my day with prayer, I'm more likely to stay centered and grounded, even when challenges arise. This connection with the Divine can be a powerful source of strength and resilience, helping you navigate the ups and downs of daily life with greater ease.

Incorporating these welcoming practices into your morning routine can transform the way you experience your day. Rather than reacting to whatever comes your way, you can approach each moment with intention and a sense of control. This proactive approach to your day is a form of self-care that pays dividends in the form of reduced stress, increased energy, and a more positive outlook on life.

Intention: Making Self-Care a Priority

The second step in the W.I.N. framework is Intention. Setting daily intentions is crucial for making room for self-care in your life. Intentions can be broken down into four key areas: mental, physical, emotional, and spiritual.

1. **Mental Intentions:** These are related to your career or purpose. One of my favorite self-care practices is keeping a daily list of commitments that never change. For example, my list includes devotion, music and movement, and reading or learning for 30 minutes. This list serves as a reminder of my priorities and helps me stay focused on what's important. Additionally, I create a daily To-Do List to help organize my tasks and reduce mental clutter. Prioritize the most important tasks and ask yourself, "What's one thing I can do today that will make everything else easier?" This is a concept I took from Gary Keller's book *The ONE Thing*. This simple practice can help you feel more in control of your day and prevent burnout.

It's also helpful to recognize that your To-Do List will never truly be complete, and that's okay. By focusing on accomplishing just 20% of your tasks each day, you can reduce the pressure you place on yourself. This approach allows you to celebrate your progress rather than feeling overwhelmed by what's left to do. Understanding that some tasks can be left for another day helps conserve your mental energy and creates a more sustainable pace.

2. **Physical Intentions:** Physical self-care is about more than just exercise. It's about listening to your body and giving it what it needs throughout the day. For example, I make it a point to get up and stretch between sessions, dance to music for a few minutes, and practice Qi Gong to balance my energy. Qi Gong is particularly beneficial because it combines physical movement with energy work, helping to release negative energy and increase positive energy in the brain and body. If you struggle with health issues or find it difficult to exercise for long periods, try breaking up your exercise into smaller chunks throughout the day. Even short bursts of movement can have a significant impact on your energy levels and overall well-being.

In addition to movement, it's important to pay attention to your nutrition. Your brain and body need proper fuel to function at their best. Skipping meals or neglecting to eat regularly can lead to low energy, mood swings, and decreased productivity. Make it a point to nourish your body with healthy foods throughout the day. Remember, self-care isn't just about what you do; it's also about what you consume. Eating balanced meals and staying hydrated are fundamental aspects of physical self-care that should not be overlooked.

3. **Emotional Intentions:** Your emotional health is just as important as your physical health. Throughout the day, take time to check in with yourself and notice how you're feeling. If you're experiencing negative emotions, acknowledge them without judgment. For example, say to yourself, "I allow myself to feel anxious, even though I don't want to feel anxious." By allowing yourself to experience your emotions, you can release them more easily and free up energy for more positive feelings. Another powerful tool is the 4-7-8 breathing technique, which involves breathing in for four counts, holding your breath for seven counts, and exhaling for eight counts. This simple practice can help reduce stress and increase relaxation by promoting the release of GABA, a calming neurotransmitter, in the brain.

Developing emotional resilience is also a key part of self-care. This involves recognizing that emotions are a natural part of the human experience and learning to navigate them in a healthy way. Journaling can be a useful practice for processing emotions and gaining insights into your feelings. By writing down your thoughts and emotions, you can gain clarity and perspective, which can help you manage your emotional state more effectively. Emotional self-care is about creating a safe space for yourself to experience and process your feelings, leading to greater emotional balance and well-being.

4. **Spiritual Intentions:** Finally, setting spiritual intentions is about connecting with something greater than yourself. Whether through prayer, meditation, or simply spending time in nature, spiritual practices can help you feel more grounded and supported. One practice I find helpful is creating a "To-Do List" for God, where I write down the things I need help with and release them to a higher power. This allows me to let go of worries and trust that everything will work out as it's meant to.

Engaging in spiritual practices can also provide a sense of purpose and direction. Whether it's through prayer, meditation, or simply reflecting on your values, spirituality can offer a deeper sense of meaning and connection in your life. It's about recognizing that you're part of something bigger and that you don't have to navigate life's challenges alone. By nurturing your spiritual self, you can cultivate a sense of peace and inner strength that supports your overall well-being.

By setting intentions in these four areas, you can create a balanced and holistic approach to self-care that supports your overall well-being.

Nighttime Rituals: Ending Your Day with Gratitude

The final step in the W.I.N. framework is Nighttime rituals. How you end your day is just as important as how you start it. Nighttime rituals can help you unwind, reflect on your day, and prepare for restful sleep.

One of my favorite nighttime rituals is practicing gratitude. Before bed, take a few moments to reflect on what went well during the day. This could be something as simple as a kind word from a friend or a task you completed. In my household, my husband and I use a method I developed called the 3x3 method. We each share three things that happened to us that were good and three things we personally did well. This practice helps us focus on the positive aspects of our day and reinforces a sense of accomplishment.

Gratitude is a powerful emotion that can transform your perspective and enhance your overall well-being. By ending your day with gratitude, you shift your focus from what went wrong to what went right, which can improve your mood and set the stage for a restful night's sleep. This practice also helps to cultivate a mindset of abundance, where you recognize and appreciate the good things in your life, no matter how small.

Another important part of my nighttime routine is cleansing, both physically and energetically. I like to take a bath with Epsom salt or use shower pods, imagining that I'm washing away the stress of the day. For highly empathetic individuals, this can be a particularly powerful practice. As you cleanse your body, you can also visualize unplugging from the energy of others and reconnecting with your soul.

It's also important to take a break from screens before bed. At least 30 to 60 minutes before you plan to sleep, put away your phone, turn off the TV, and give your brain time to wind down. Bedtime rituals help signal to your brain that it's time to rest, leading to better sleep and overall health.

Lastly, consider creating a bedtime routine that includes relaxation techniques such as reading, listening to calming music, or practicing deep breathing exercises. These activities can help you transition from the busyness of the day to a state of relaxation, making it easier to fall and stay asleep. Prioritizing sleep as a key component of self-care is essential for maintaining your health and well-being.

Conclusion: Making Self-Care a Daily Priority

Self-care should be a top priority for everyone because when you don't take care of yourself, your health—and, by extension, your ability to care for others—suffers. My own experience has shown me that neglecting self-care can have serious consequences. That's why I now emphasize the importance of daily self-care to everyone I work with, no matter what they're going through. By taking a holistic approach to self-care and incorporating it into your daily routine, you can improve your energy levels, mental health, and overall well-being.

Remember, self-care doesn't have to be complicated or time-consuming. The W.I.N. framework offers a simple and effective way to make self-care a part of your everyday life. By Welcoming the day with positivity, setting Intentions for your mental, physical, emotional, and spiritual well-being, and ending the day with Nighttime rituals that promote relaxation and gratitude, you can create a life where you consistently W.I.N. at self-care.

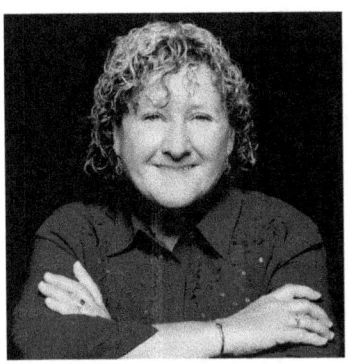

Julie Ashlock

Jules Body Shoppe
CMHC, CMCS, CPT, LMT

https://www.linkedin.com/in/julieashlock/
https://www.facebook.com/jbodyshoppe
https://www.instagram.com/julesbodyshoppe
https://julesbodyshoppe.com
https://julesbodyshoppe.idlife.com

Julie Ashlock aka "Jules" is a Certified Master Health Coach, Certified Menopause Coaching Specialist, Certified Nutritionist, and Certified Personal Trainer with over 16 years experience in the health and wellness industry. Passionate about empowering women to seek root cause solutions to their health challenges and concerns, Jules tailors wellness plans based on your DNA and lifestyle. She takes the guesswork out of how you eat, exercise and supplement. Knowing that one size does not fit all, Jules takes a unique approach that integrates DNA testing, detoxing and customized nutrition and creates an individualized plan to have every client feeling their absolute best. Jules' personal journey regarding her MTHFR (methylenetetrahydrofolate reductase) gene variants has been transformative, enabling her to manage her own health journey with excellence and uninterrupted vitality. She is dedicated to helping others to feel seen, heard and understood so that they can not only heal themselves, but their future generations to come.

Unlocking Your Genetic Code: The MTHFR Gene's Hidden Secrets

By Julie Ashlock

Have you ever wondered why health just doesn't seem to come easy for some, despite their best efforts? For many, the answer lies hidden in their DNA. Understanding the MTHFR gene and its variants can be a key to unlocking better health and well-being. Imagine discovering a piece of your genetic puzzle that could explain persistent fatigue, mood swings, or even heart health issues. By knowing your MTHFR status, you are taking an empowering step towards a more personalized approach to health. This chapter will guide you through the significance of the MTHFR gene, helping you to connect the dots and potentially transform your health journey.

Let's discuss what MTHFR is exactly. The MTHFR gene (Methylenetetrahydrofolate Reductase) is a gene that provides instructions for making an enzyme that plays a crucial role in processing amino acids, the building blocks of proteins. This enzyme is particularly important for a chemical reaction involving forms of the vitamin folate (also called vitamin B9) and the conversion of the amino acid homocysteine to methionine, which is used by the body to make proteins and other important compounds.

There are three main MTHFR gene variants. The C677T Variant (rs1801133) is the most studied MTHFR gene variant. When an individual is homozygous for C677T (having two copies), it is associated with reduced enzyme activity and higher homocysteine levels, which may increase the risk of cardiovascular diseases, neural tube defects, and other health issues. In the case of being heterozygous (having one copy), the impact is lesser but can still influence overall health.

The A1298C Variant (rs1801131) is another common variant. Being homozygous for A1298C (having two copies) is linked to reduced enzyme efficiency and various health complications, although these are typically less severe than those associated with the C677T variant. If one is heterozygous for A1298C (having one copy), there might be a moderate effect on enzyme function.

Having Combined Heterozygosity (one copy of each mutation for C677T & A1298C) can similarly reduce enzyme activity and increase health risks related to elevated homocysteine levels.

For individuals with the Normal/Non-Mutation (Wild-Type), there is no mutation present in the MTHFR gene. This results in normal enzyme activity and typical processing of folate and homocysteine, without increased health risks related to the MTHFR gene.

It is estimated that nearly 40% of the population has at least one of these variants.

The MTHFR gene functions primarily in folate metabolism and homocysteine regulation. The enzyme produced by the MTHFR gene is vital for converting 5,10-methylenetetrahydrofolate to 5-methyltetrahydrofolate, an essential step in converting the amino acid homocysteine to methionine. Proper functioning of the MTHFR gene helps maintain balanced levels of homocysteine, an amino acid that can be harmful at elevated levels.

Why should you be concerned about having an MTHFR gene variant(s)? When I first learned about MTHFR mutations, I was surprised to discover how profoundly they can impact various aspects of health. Living with a variant of the MTHFR gene can sometimes feel like navigating a labyrinth of health challenges. For many, it begins with a pervasive sense of fatigue and weakness that can deflate daily vibrancy and enthusiasm. Mental health can also be impacted, with conditions, such as depression, anxiety, and bipolar disorder casting long shadows on emotional well-being. Cardiovascular problems, including high blood pressure, elevated homocysteine levels, and an increased risk of blood clots, add another layer of concern.

For those dreaming of starting or expanding their families, recurrent miscarriages and fertility issues can be especially heartbreaking. Neurological problems, such as migraines, memory loss, and neuropathy, might manifest, while chronic pain conditions, including muscle and joint pain or fibromyalgia, create constant discomfort. The risk of birth defects, such as neural tube defects like spina bifida in offspring, adds a further dimension of worry. Digestive disorders like irritable bowel syndrome (IBS), hormonal imbalances including irregular menstrual cycles and polycystic ovary syndrome (PCOS), and autoimmune diseases like rheumatoid arthritis or fibromyalgia can also be part of the complex picture. Even developmental disorders such as ADHD and developmental delays in children are linked to MTHFR variants.

It's important to remember, however, that not everyone with an MTHFR variant will face these issues. Your unique genetic predisposition, lifestyle choices, and environmental factors all intersect to shape your health journey. Embracing this knowledge empowers you to take proactive steps tailored to your individual needs, fostering hope and resilience along the way. Knowing this, one feels an even greater urgency to understand our genetic blueprint, doesn't it?

Understanding the intricacies of your genetic makeup can feel overwhelming, yet the value of genetic testing for MTHFR mutations cannot be overstated. By identifying specific mutations such as C677T and A1298C in the MTHFR gene, these tests can reveal vital insights into how well your enzyme functions. Knowing your MTHFR status opens the door to personalized solutions, where dietary and supplement recommendations—like increasing your methylated folate intake—can be fine-tuned to suit your unique needs. This isn't just about optimizing daily nutrition; it's about taking proactive steps for your long-term health. For those planning a family, such genetic information becomes even more critical, serving as a guide for precautions that can safeguard both mother and baby. It's empowering to know that through understanding your genetic blueprint, you can take targeted actions to enhance your well-being and the health of your loved ones.

Knowledge and awareness are vitally important, but what's more important is taking the next step—finding out if you are part of the 40% affected by one or more of these variants, and getting the absolute best, pharmaceutical-grade nutritional supplementation into your system that addresses the root cause and truly helps to alleviate your health challenges. Find out more information here: https://julesbodyshoppe.idlife.com/shop/product/05-0033.

You don't need to keep guessing why you aren't feeling your absolute best self anymore—you owe it to yourself to get to the root cause of your health challenges and take steps to live your best life!

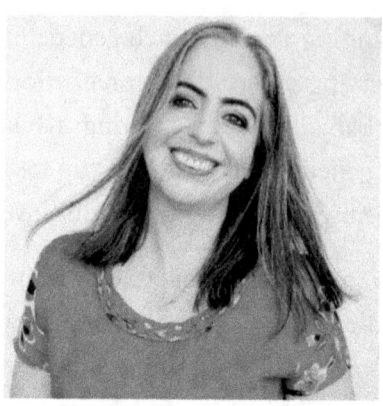

Dr. Teresa Ibarra

CEO of Heal and Thrive Coaching

https://www.linkedin.com/in/dr-teresa-ibarra/
https://www.facebook.com/teresa.ibarra.796/
https://www.instagram.com/drteresaibarra/
https://www.drteresa.com.au/
http://www.themetabolicmagic.com/

Dr. Teresa Ibarra is a dedicated holistic health coach specializing in empowering women to reverse autoimmune diseases through natural methods. With expertise in fasting, mind-body connection, Iridology, and energy healing, Dr. Ibarra offers a comprehensive approach to wellness. Her personal journey from being told she'd need lifelong medication to successfully reversing her autoimmune condition serves as a powerful testament to her methods. Passionate about helping others achieve similar transformations, Dr. Ibarra combines her professional knowledge with her own lived experience to inspire and guide women toward vibrant health and vitality.

Awaken Your Inner Healer: A Story of Hope and Transformation

By Dr. Teresa Ibarra

When I was diagnosed with Graves' disease, my world came to a standstill. The doctors told me my immune system was attacking my thyroid and that there was no option other than to take medication for the rest of my life. "There's nothing you can do," they said. My body, they explained, was turning against me. As I left the doctor's office with a prescription in hand and a heart heavy with fear, anger, and hopelessness, I couldn't accept that this was my future.

I was consumed with questions: *Why is this happening to me? Why is my body failing me?* But deep inside, there was a small, unwavering voice. It whispered: *Your body is a miracle.* I knew, intuitively, that something was out of balance, and I was determined to uncover what I had done to contribute to this illness. Instead of accepting a future dictated by medication, I made a conscious decision to take control of my health. That choice marked the beginning of my journey into healing, transformation, and empowerment.

The Moment of Awakening

When the initial shock of the diagnosis subsided, I reflected on the years leading up to that moment. It became clear that my body had been crying out for help long before Graves' disease was diagnosed. I remembered the frequent migraines that left me incapacitated, the eczema that flared up unexpectedly, and the digestive issues that had plagued me for years. I had normalized these symptoms, brushing them off as minor inconveniences in my busy life, failing to truly listen to what my body was telling me.

But now, I couldn't ignore the signs any longer. My body was screaming for attention, and I finally decided to listen.

Detoxing Body and Soul

The first step in my healing journey was detoxification—not just of my body, but of my entire environment. I knew instinctively that what I was consuming was affecting my health, but I also realized that the toxins surrounding me were just as harmful. I began by cleaning up my diet, eliminating processed foods, sugars, and harmful chemicals. I switched to organic, whole foods and hydrated my body with clean, purified water.

But I didn't stop there. I took a hard look at my home environment, removing toxic household cleaners, personal care products, and anything that might be adding to my body's toxic load. I also began to recognize the need for emotional detox. Years of suppressed emotions—fear, resentment, anger, and sadness—had been stored within me, contributing to the disease. I turned to practices such as journaling, meditation, and breathwork to help release these long-held emotions. Finally, confronting these feelings felt liberating and essential to my healing.

Healing Through the Subconscious Mind

As I continued my journey, I realized that true healing went beyond the physical. I began studying the subconscious mind, learning how deeply our beliefs, thoughts, and emotions affect our health. For years, I had been operating from a place of fear, stress, and self-doubt. These unconscious patterns had driven my body into a state of imbalance, further fueling my disease.

I made the decision to shift my mindset and consciously create the reality I desired. I used visualization techniques and positive affirmations to reprogram my mind. Every day, I visualized myself as healthy, vibrant, and full of energy. I affirmed that my body was capable of healing itself, and slowly but surely, I began to believe it with every fiber of my being. I no longer viewed my body as something that had betrayed me, but rather as a miraculous system designed to heal and thrive.

Tapping Into Energy Healing

I had always known about the energy body, even from a young age. I could sense the subtle vibrations within and around me, and I felt deeply connected to the idea that we are more than just our physical selves. However, it wasn't until my health crisis with Graves' disease that I fully embraced the power of energy healing and experienced its transformative potential.

As part of my healing process, I began to explore energy practices like chakra balancing, reiki, and other forms of energy work. These techniques were designed to clear and align the body's energy systems, and I quickly realized that emotional trauma, limiting beliefs, and external stressors had been disrupting the flow of energy within me for years. By working with my energy, I began to release old patterns that were holding me back and contributing to my illness.

Through energy healing, I learned to let go of fear, anger, and emotional traumas that had been stored in my energetic field. With each session, it felt as though my cells were being recharged, and my entire system was coming back into balance. The more I worked with energy, the more my physical body began to heal. This process was profound. It wasn't just a theory; I experienced firsthand how my health shifted as I aligned with my energy body.

Symptoms that had once plagued me—migraines, eczema, digestive issues—started to fade. My thyroid function began to return to normal. I discovered that energy healing wasn't just a tool for recovery; it was a way to realign my body and mind with their innate wisdom and potential for self-healing.

Understanding the Warning Signs

As I healed, I gained a profound understanding of my body's earlier cries for help. Those years of migraines, skin flare-ups, and digestive issues were not random; they were warning signs that something was out of alignment. My immune system had become confused and overactive because I had not been listening to my body's signals. Once I began addressing the root causes—both physical and emotional—my body responded with healing and vitality.

Empowering Others

Reversing my autoimmune disease was a life-changing experience, one that gave me back my health, my energy, and my hope. But more importantly, it empowered me to help others on their own healing journeys. Graves' disease wasn't my enemy; it was my body's way of alerting me to the deeper imbalances I had been ignoring for years.

Now, I dedicate my life to guiding others through their healing processes. I want women to know that their bodies are not broken, and their diagnoses are not life sentences. With the right tools, mindset, and support, healing is possible. I am living proof of that.

Healing is not just about addressing symptoms; it's about understanding the deeper layers of what's going on in the body, mind, and energy system. When we awaken to our inner healer, we unlock the codes to a life of wholeness, vitality, and peace. My hope is that my story will inspire you to listen to your body, trust in its wisdom, and take the steps necessary to reclaim your health.

You, too, can awaken your inner healer. Your body is a miracle, and it is always working in your favor.

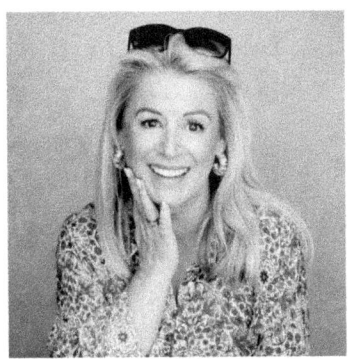

Jane Butler

Founder and CEO of Individually You Coaching
Womens Health and Wellness Coach,

https://www.facebook.com/groups/loveyourmenopausewithjane/
https://www.instagram.com/individually.you/
http://www.individuallyyoucoaching.com/
http://www.aloeshopwithjane.com/

Jane Butler, MSc, is a former UK Registered Nurse and Consultant Nurse for Heart Failure with over 4 decades of experience in the NHS. Now a certified Health Coach specializing in women's health, Jane is a dedicated advocate for menopause awareness, empowering women with the latest information and support. She is the founder and CEO of "Individually You Coaching," offering personalized lifestyle approaches to help women thrive in the next chapter of their lives. Having experienced insomnia during her own menopause transition, Jane is passionate about helping women overcome sleep problems. She embraces a "back to basics" approach to problem-solving as the foundation of her coaching methodology. Jane balances her professional passion with her roles as a wife, mother, and grandmother, and she splits her time between the UK and California. Her interests include cooking, reading, traveling and family. Join her in her "Love your menopause with Jane" Facebook group.

The Glow Trio

By Jane Butler

In the bustling chaos of midlife, where responsibilities stack up like dishes after a family dinner, finding time for yourself can feel impossible. As a former registered nurse and now a dedicated women's health coach, I've seen the transformative power of the simple yet profoundly effective trio: sleep, nutrition, and exercise. These elements are not just about living longer but about living better, glowing from the inside out.

Sleep

Let's start with sleep, the often-overlooked hero in our quest for well-being. As a nurse, I witnessed firsthand the toll that poor sleep can take on the body and mind. Sleep deprivation was often at the root of many chronic conditions I treated, from hypertension to depression. I remember one patient, let's call her Linda, who was a classic case. She was a mid-aged woman juggling a demanding job, teenage kids, and aging parents. Linda prided herself on needing only four hours of sleep to function. But as she approached her late 40s, her energy plummeted, she gained weight, and her once radiant skin dulled.

Linda's story is not unique. We live in a culture that celebrates busyness, often at the expense of our well-being. But here's the truth: Sleep is not a luxury; it's a necessity. During sleep, our bodies perform critical maintenance work—repairing cells, balancing hormones, and consolidating memories. For women in mid-age, quality sleep is even more crucial. As we age, our bodies produce less of the growth hormone that helps to repair and rejuvenate our skin. Sleep is the time when this process happens most effectively. Missing out on sleep means missing out on that vital repair work, leading to premature aging, a sluggish metabolism, and a diminished immune system.

In my own journey, sleep was the first area I had to reevaluate. Transitioning from a nurse to a health coach meant I had to practice what I preached. I used to survive on five to six hours of sleep, convincing myself that it was enough. But as I entered my mid-40s, I noticed I was more irritable and less focused, and my skin started showing signs of stress. It was then that I made sleep a priority. I began creating a bedtime routine that included shutting off screens an hour before bed, practicing deep breathing exercises, and making my bedroom a sanctuary—cool, dark, and quiet. The difference was remarkable. Not only did I feel more energized, but I also noticed my skin looking more vibrant, and my mood improved significantly.

Nutrition

Nutrition is the second cornerstone of the glow trio. As a nurse, I was always aware of the importance of a balanced diet, but it wasn't until I started coaching that I truly understood how deeply nutrition affects every aspect of our health. The food we eat fuels our bodies, and more importantly, it fuels our glow. For women in mid-age, this is particularly critical because our nutritional needs change as we age.

One amusing story that sticks with me is from a client, Sarah, who was obsessed with finding the "perfect" anti-aging cream. She spent a small fortune on every product that promised to turn back the clock, yet she continued to eat processed foods, skip meals, and drink water minimally. Her skin was dull, and she was constantly fatigued. We started with a simple change—adding more fresh vegetables, lean proteins, and healthy fats to her diet, and drastically reducing sugar. Within weeks, Sarah's skin began to glow, her energy levels skyrocketed, and she even shed a few pounds without trying. She finally realized that no cream could replace the benefits of nourishing her body from the inside out.

For women in mid-age, the focus should be on foods rich in antioxidants, vitamins, and minerals that support skin health, energy levels, and hormonal balance. Think colorful fruits and vegetables, nuts, seeds, lean proteins, and whole grains. Omega-3 fatty acids, found in foods like salmon, flaxseeds, and walnuts, are particularly beneficial as they help maintain skin elasticity and hydration. Hydration is another key aspect—drinking enough water keeps the skin plump and flushes out toxins, giving you that youthful glow.

I always tell my clients that every meal is an opportunity to nourish their bodies. When you start seeing food as fuel, you begin to make choices that not only taste good but also make you feel good. And when you feel good on the inside, it radiates on the outside.

Exercising

Last but certainly not least, let's talk about exercise. Exercise is often seen as a means to an end—primarily weight loss. But the benefits of regular physical activity go far beyond fitting into a smaller dress size. For women in mid-age, exercise is a powerful tool to combat the effects of aging, improve mental health, and, yes, keep that glow alive.

I vividly remember a client, Julie, who came to me with a singular goal: to lose 20 pounds before her 50th birthday. She dreaded exercise and had tried every fad diet out there. We started small, integrating short walks into her day and gradually introducing strength training. Julie was surprised to find that not only did she start losing weight, but her energy levels soared, and she felt more confident. The best part? Julie began to enjoy exercise. It became her "me time," a way to relieve stress and reconnect with herself.

Exercise helps regulate hormones, which is crucial as we age and our bodies undergo various changes. Regular physical activity boosts endorphins, the body's natural mood lifters, helping to combat anxiety and depression, which can be more prevalent during mid-age. Strength training, in particular, is vital for women as it helps to maintain muscle mass, increase metabolism, and improve bone density, reducing the risk of osteoporosis. Even something as simple as a daily walk can improve circulation, delivering more oxygen and nutrients to the skin, which contributes to that radiant glow.

In my journey from nursing to coaching, I learned to embrace exercise not just as a health necessity but as a way to celebrate what my body could do. It's not about punishing yourself in the gym; it's about moving in ways that make you feel alive. Whether it's dancing in your living room, hiking in nature, or practicing yoga, find what you love and do it regularly.

Conclusion

As we reach mid-age, it's easy to get caught up in the idea that aging is something to be feared or fought against. But I've learned, both through my own experiences and those of the women I've worked with, that aging can be a beautiful journey. It's a time to focus on what truly matters—taking care of our bodies, minds, and spirits so that we can continue to shine brightly in the years to come.

The glow that we seek isn't found in a bottle or a fad diet; it's cultivated through good sleep, nourishing food, and regular exercise. These are the foundational elements that support our health, vitality, and confidence. As a former nurse and now a women's health coach, I've seen how transformative these practices can be.

So, embrace sleep as your nightly reset, choose foods that nourish and energize you, and move your body in ways that make you feel strong and joyful. These are the keys to glowing from the inside out, to being the vibrant, radiant woman you were always meant to be.

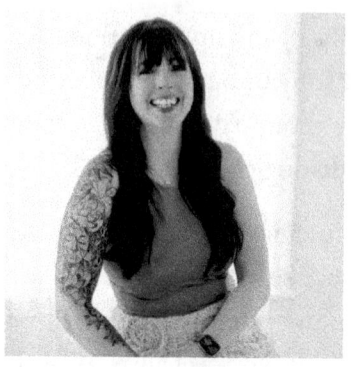

Jacquelyn Rodriguez

Founder and CEO of Enlightened Styles

https://www.linkedin.com/in/cleanbeautybizcoach/
https://www.facebook.com/CleanBeautyBizCoach
https://www.instagram.com/cleanbeautybizcoach/
https://www.cleanbeautybiz.com/
https://www.enlightenedstyles.com/

Jacquelyn is an accomplished beauty industry expert, holistic salon owner, and advocate for clean, sustainable, and conscious beauty practices. With over 26 years of experience as a cosmetologist and salon owner, she founded Enlightened Styles, a pioneering salon that integrates holistic and eco-conscious services into the beauty experience. Jacquelyn is also the co-founder of the nonprofit Green Beauty Community, where she supports salon owners in transitioning to clean, sustainable business models. Passionate about education and mentorship, she launched the Holistic Salon Academy to empower salon owners with the knowledge and tools to implement sustainable and holistic practices in their own businesses. Beyond the salon, Jacquelyn speaks at industry events and hosts a podcast that challenges beauty industry norms, promoting sustainability and wellness. Her journey of personal transformation drives her mission to inspire others to embrace wellness, advocate for clean beauty, and radiate confidence from the inside out.

Advocate for Yourself: The Power of Conscious Choices

By Jacquelyn Rodriguez

Our culture is always trying to tell us how we should act, what we should buy, and how we should see beauty. The pressure to always be one step ahead, pursue perfection, and become engrossed in the latest trends is real. But what if we took a step back and began to question everything? What if, rather than conforming to society's expectations, we prioritized decisions that reflected our beliefs, our health, and the kind of future we envisioned for ourselves?

That's where advocating for yourself comes in. It's not just about speaking up; it's about recognizing your worth and making conscious decisions that reflect that understanding. It's about asking, "Is this really good for me? Is it healthy for my family and the planet?" The moment you start asking these questions, you take back your power and step into a more aligned life.

I know how easy it is to get swept up in the beauty standards society imposes. I didn't grow up feeling beautiful. I spent years trying to fit into the mold society created, hoping I could become what everyone else seemed to expect. As a cosmetologist, I helped others feel beautiful, but inside, I struggled with the same insecurities. It wasn't until I became a mother that I started to see things differently. Everything changed when I realized beauty is about making choices that serve you.

I'll never forget the moment that set me on this path. I was cleaning the bathroom, trying to keep my toddlers out because I didn't want them breathing in the fumes from the cleaning products. That's when it hit me: if I didn't want my kids breathing this in, why was I? That moment was a wake-up call. I started researching what was in the products we used daily, from cleaners to shampoos and makeup. What I found was shocking. We were surrounded by toxins.

This discovery pushed me to make changes. But I didn't overhaul everything overnight, and neither do you. Change happens step by step, through small, conscious decisions. When my shampoo ran out, I found a cleaner alternative. When my lotion was used up, I looked for a healthier option. Each small decision led my family and me toward a cleaner lifestyle.

This journey isn't about reaching an impossible standard. It's about giving yourself permission to question the products, services, and businesses you support. Are they aligned with your values? Are they good for you, your family, and the environment? You don't need permission to ask these questions, but sometimes, we need a reminder that it's okay to start.

The next time you run out of a product, pause before buying the same brand. Ask yourself: "Is this product still working for me? Is it healthy? Does the company behind it reflect my values?" If the answer is no, explore better options. With so many brands committed to transparency and sustainability, it's easier to make choices that are good for your health and the planet.

As I navigated this journey, I realized it wasn't just about my family or business—it was about being part of something bigger. When we, as consumers, demand better products and services, we help create lasting change. Large corporations seem powerful, but they rely on us. When we stop supporting brands that don't align with our values, they're forced to shift. A small decision can make a big impact.

You don't have to tackle everything at once. The goal is not to overwhelm yourself but to empower you to make decisions that feel right. It's okay if you're the only one in your circle making these changes. I've been there. People might think you're crazy, but they're watching. Eventually, they may follow your lead.

For me, it started with cleaning products, but the mindset shift extended to every part of my life—from the products I used in my salon to personal care items and the businesses I supported. Each small change created a ripple effect that improved my health and made me feel more empowered and aligned with my values.

As I continue on this path, I've seen how these small steps can transform not just my life, but the lives of those around me. You become part of a movement—a collective of people choosing better, healthier, more conscious options. And that's powerful.

Advocating for yourself means standing up for your health, your family, and the planet. It means choosing products and services that reflect what you believe in. You deserve to feel good about the choices you make and to live a life aligned with your values. This journey isn't about guilt or judgment. You're not here to push your choices on others. You're leading by example. As you live out your values, people will start to notice and ask questions. That's when real change begins.

The beauty of this journey is that it doesn't have to be overwhelming. You can start small. The next time you're about to buy something, research cleaner options. Use apps or websites to check ingredients and learn about the companies behind the products. Are they committed to transparency and sustainability, or are they just using buzzwords? Look for brands that align with your values.

Remember, this isn't about perfection. It's okay to take your time, to make mistakes, and to keep learning. Every conscious decision you make is a step toward a healthier, more aligned life—for you, your family, and the planet.

Most importantly, you are worthy of making these choices. You deserve to live a life that's healthy, conscious, and aligned with your values. When enough of us make these small choices, the ripple effect will create a positive impact on the world around us. And that's the power of advocating for yourself—it's not just about you; it's about the change we create together.

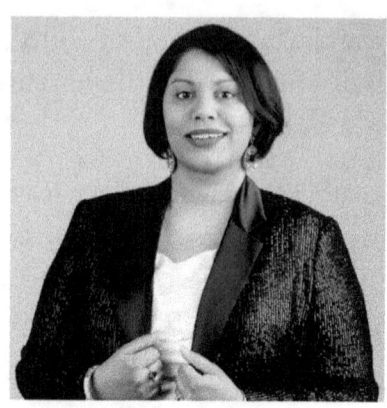

Tina Salmon

Founder and CEO of Coachanizer
Business & Burnout Management Coach

https://www.linkedin.com/in/tina-salmon/
https://www.facebook.com/Coachanizer
https://www.instagram.com/coachanizer/
https://www.thecoachanizer.com/

Tina Salmon, LCSW, MPA, CCM, is a Business Burnout Management Coach, Licensed Psychotherapist, NLP Integrative Practitioner, Speaker, and CEO of Coachanizer. With over 20 years of experience in clinical and business settings, Tina helps high-performing leaders thrive without sacrificing their health. She is known for her neuroscience-backed strategies that empower clients to reclaim their time, prevent burnout, and achieve lasting fulfillment in both their careers and personal lives.

Tina's expertise in mental health, applied neuroscience, and business wellness coaching provides transformative insights for a healthier, more integrative life. Having served over 5,000 clients and completed more than 20,000 individual sessions, Tina is a leading authority in therapeutic practice and business strategy. She continues to inspire others to find greater personal fulfillment while maintaining professional success.

From Tragedy to Triumph: Embracing Your Healthy Glow

By Tina Salmon

I was born on the Caribbean island of Trinidad, and my life was shaped by tragedy early on. At just three months old, my father, only 23, was struck by lightning while fishing and passed away. His sudden death ingrained in me a belief that life was short and time was fleeting. Growing up, I felt a constant urgency to accelerate everything.

Fast forward to 2020, at the height of the pandemic, when life hit hard again. I lost my father's only brother, contracted COVID-19, and faced an overwhelming workload in my 9-5 job while trying to grow my business. The balance between work, maintaining my marriage, and simply staying afloat felt impossible. I was overwhelmed, overworked, and trapped in a cycle of stress and exhaustion.

I started getting frequent headaches, struggled with sleep, and couldn't shut off my thoughts—even on date nights, my mind was consumed by the business. My body began to send out warning signs: mental exhaustion, physical fatigue, and random electric shocks. Yet, like many high achievers, I believed that perseverance was the key to success, so I pushed through.

I did what most people do when overwhelmed, I tried to escape through distractions. I shopped online, booked spa days, indulged in wine tours, and downloaded another time management app. But none of these quick fixes worked. Eventually, I went to my primary care doctor, who found nothing wrong. I saw a neurologist who, after less than 10 minutes, prescribed medication with harsh side effects.

Finally, I found a cardiologist who took the time to listen. After thorough conversations and testing, he suggested I might be experiencing burnout and encouraged me to address the root causes of my stress. Extensive research confirmed I was suffering from anxiety jolts, where the body reacts to extreme stress.

This diagnosis forced me to make a tough decision: keep spinning my wheels or focus on my health. I chose the latter, taking a six-month leave from work and pressing pause on growing my business. My healing journey began with basic self-care eating healthy, drinking more water, exercising, spending time with loved ones, and seeking therapy to process the grief of losing my dad and uncle.

These actions helped restore my physical and mental health, but I quickly realized that life's stressors would always be present. What mattered was how I responded to them rather than staying in constant reaction mode. Reflecting on my past, I understood that losing my father and being raised to be a high achiever had shaped my beliefs about time and success. I worked relentlessly because I believed life was short, but that mindset led to burnout.

As I processed my experiences, I realized that my father lived his life fully, and I needed to do the same. I learned to cherish moments, take care of myself, and be present in my most important relationships while growing a business that brought me joy. I came to understand that while stress is inevitable, how we perceive and manage it is what truly defines our experience.

This journey led me to realize the importance of an unshakeable mindset. I became a certified transformational mindset coach, and my curiosity about the brain led me to pursue certifications in applied neuroscience and neuro-linguistic programming. Combining 20 years of experience in mental health, I developed the S.A.F.E. Methodology, a structured approach that empowers individuals to prevent burnout by prioritizing wellness and balancing busy lives.

If you or someone you know is experiencing burnout, the first step is stabilizing the body—consult a medical provider to rule out any underlying conditions. Next, clarify your vision and align your daily habits with that vision. Often, we get so caught up in doing everything for everyone else that we lose sight of our own goals. As you implement your plan, you'll encounter opportunities to break free from limiting beliefs about time, money, and relationships. This is the most crucial phase of the journey and where I focus much of my work with clients. Addressing the root causes of stress enables us to make new, empowering decisions that rewire our brains and accelerate results.

Through my coaching practice, I share the lessons I've learned to help others achieve sustainable success. It's not just about avoiding burnout—it's about creating a life where professional achievement and personal well-being coexist. With the right mindset, you can find balance and thrive in all areas of life. By sharing my journey, I hope to inspire others to find joy, success, and fulfillment in both their personal and professional lives.

As you reflect on your own journey, I invite you to take the first step toward embracing your healthy glow. Ask yourself: What's your body telling you right now? Are you feeling overwhelmed, exhausted, or a bit unfulfilled? It's time to pause, reassess, and take action.

Consider scheduling a consultation with a health professional to explore any underlying issues that may be impacting your well-being. Next, take a moment to clarify your vision for a fulfilling life. What are your core values? What truly matters to you? Align your daily habits with that vision and commit to putting your health and happiness first.

If you're ready to dig deeper and transform how you approach life and work, let's connect! I would love to explore the S.A.F.E. Methodology with you. Together, we can tackle those limiting beliefs and build a mindset that empowers you to thrive.

Don't let burnout dictate your life. Take charge of your health, reclaim your time, and step into a new chapter filled with joy and sustainable success. Remember, you are not alone in this journey; you have the power to rise from tragedy to triumph. Your healthy glow awaits, embrace it!

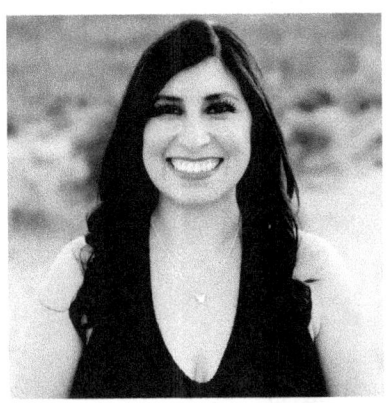

Ana Lucia Martinez, RN

A New Adventure
Peer to Peer Mentor

https://www.linkedin.com/in/anamlv
https://www.facebook.com/anarnclc
https://www.instagram.com/anam.rnclc/
https://www.fearlessmotherhoodjourney.com
https://calendly.com/anamlv/30min

Ana is a homeschooling mom of three daughters and a versatile professional. As a Registered Nurse, Certified Lactation Counselor, Cruise Planners Travel Specialist, HowMoneyWorks Financial Educator, and author, she has built a diverse career. Ana graduated from the University of Nevada, Las Vegas, in 2013 with a Bachelor of Science in Nursing, gaining experience in various specialties, including labor, delivery, postpartum, and hospice care.

In 2017, she expanded her role as a Certified Lactation Counselor, and in 2022, driven by her passion for travel, she became a Travel Specialist. By 2024, Ana embraced entrepreneurship in the financial industry and began her writing journey, while continuing her previous work.

In her free time, Ana enjoys dancing and is currently traveling full-time with her family in an RV. She believes life is too short to settle for anything less than extraordinary, especially when it comes to living authentically as your true self.

Crafting Your Labor of Love: The Power of Informed Choices and Preparation

By Ana Lucia Martinez, RN

As young girls, we often played with dolls, pretending to be mothers nurturing and feeding our cherished toys. However, I did not truly consider how I would deliver my own babies once I was old enough to understand the process. My focus was more on avoiding pregnancy and figuring out which birth control would be most effective. How did you envision the experience of delivering your babies?

It wasn't until I became pregnant and my former husband asked me what I was going to do for pain management during labor that I started to consider any alternatives. My understanding of childbirth at the time came from what I observed in nursing school during my obstetric rotation, and both vaginal delivery and C-sections seemed painful, scary, and just awful. Still, I told my former husband that if we could research and find an alternative, I would be open to giving it a chance.

We were blessed to go on a babymoon cruise where we met a couple at dinner. We mentioned my pregnancy, and they told us about The Bradley Method®. Once home, we Googled it and were thrilled to find a teacher right in our hometown of Las Vegas, Nevada!

The Bradley Method® is a 12-week childbirth education course that is unique in its approach. As stated on their website, "[Their] classes stress the importance of Healthy Baby, Healthy Mother, and Healthy Families. [They] attract Families who are willing to take the responsibility needed for preparation and birth" (The Bradley Method 2024, *Why take classes in The Bradley Method® of natural childbirth?*, accessed 20 October 2024, <https://bradleybirth.com/WhyBradley.aspx>). The program teaches expecting parents about their choices during pregnancy, labor, delivery, and postpartum. It emphasizes mental, emotional, and physical wellness and relaxation, which can help keep the pregnant person low-risk.

In class, we watched videos of families using The Bradley Method® in various settings, including hospitals, birthing centers, and at home. This was my first exposure to the concept of homebirth. I had no idea I even had options when it came to choosing where to deliver my baby. Where would you feel most safe bringing your little one into the world?

For the first time in my life, I felt empowered. I was taking responsibility for the birth of my baby and truly doing something I wanted to do. The Bradley Method® helped me build confidence from the inside out, enabling me to make informed choices and prepare for the birth I desired.

During my pregnancy, I remained low-risk until I tested positive for group beta strep (GBS). That is when we decided to switch to a homebirth. The obstetrician informed us that if I didn't receive the standard protocol of two rounds of antibiotics during labor, our baby would be taken away to the neonatal intensive care unit (NICU) for observation. How dare he threaten us like that! We were furious at our obstetrician, and that was the final push we needed to choose a homebirth.

With the help of our Bradley teacher, we found a Certified Professional Midwife (CPM) we trusted, albeit very late in pregnancy. We paid out of pocket for the homebirth, as no health insurance in Nevada covers it, but it was the best money we spent. My only regret was not having our midwife sooner to help us prepare for what lay ahead. That is why, for my subsequent two pregnancies, I was fortunate to work with the same midwifery team from the beginning, ensuring the safe home births of my daughters.

As a wonderful bonus, my daughters were involved and present for the births of their sisters, which was truly priceless. Who would you want to be involved in your births?

Furthermore, based on my personal and professional experience as a labor, delivery, and postpartum nurse, I arrived at two key observations:

1. Many women choose to remain unprepared and uninformed about the choices they need to make, often leaving the responsibility to their medical team. Unfortunately, labor, delivery, and the postpartum period inevitably involve pain—whether physical, mental, or emotional. Modern society complicates this further; it often fails to understand maternity, as evidenced by our mortality rates, and many women do not maintain active lifestyles that support childbirth. Consequently, trying to "wing it" or relying on the idea that "ignorance is bliss" is not effective, especially when information is so readily available online.

2. We typically don't see, care about, or discuss motherhood until it is our turn to become a mother. As Julia Jones, founding director of Newborn Mothers, a postpartum educator and best-selling author, notes, "When a baby is born, so is a mother...and the birth of a mother can be more intense than childbirth" (accessed 20 October 2024, <https://newbornmothers.com/>). When we lack the opportunity to witness our mothers, aunts, cousins, or others giving birth—often a private experience behind closed doors in hospitals—we miss the chance to be prepared for what lies ahead. Usually, unsolicited advice replaces the practical tips and support that a newborn mother truly needs to maintain her sanity during this challenging season. It often feels like women hesitate to discuss the realities of transitioning into motherhood, parenting, and relationships. There's also a reluctance to acknowledge the grief that can accompany the shift from being a woman to becoming a mother, or to be nonjudgmental about the parenting choices made by others.

To be clear, I understand that every birth and situation is different. However, I also know that without the education and preparation I gained from The Bradley Method® and my midwifery team, I would not have learned the skills necessary to achieve the births I desired for myself and my daughters. In life, learning and mastering a skill takes practice and time.

Moreover, while I personally prefer The Bradley Method®, there are numerous other approaches to preparing for labor and parenting. Today, with the wealth of information available online, along with resources like social media and the support of doulas, you have many options to explore.

For these reasons, I want to emphasize that you have the **CHOICE** to **PREPARE** and find **SUPPORT**. You have the choice to educate yourself, to prepare for labor and birth, and to seek support—whether paid or unpaid—for yourself and your family.

Would you sign up for a marathon in nine months and just show up? No, a typical person would prepare. You would train physically, mentally, and emotionally. You would turn to Google and YouTube or ask friends and family if they've run a marathon or know someone who has, seeking their advice. Labor can be comparable to hiking 50 miles! It's called labor for a reason—your body is working hard.

Stay active! Build your stamina! Take action! Enroll in classes and learn. What can you do to keep moving? Pregnancy is not the time to be sedentary. *Disclaimer: Listen to your body and consult your provider.*

Equally important is finding the support you need for yourself and your family. The day a baby is born, so is a mother. While people are eager to hold the baby, who is there to care for the mother? This is where my passion for supporting families during pregnancy, labor and delivery, postpartum, and lactation began. I felt anxious, lonely, and overwhelmed. I was told that I hadn't asked for help the first time, so I made sure to reach out for support with my second. Yet, I received little to no assistance from family and friends, and the pandemic only exacerbated the situation. No mother or family should feel anxious, lonely, or overwhelmed.

With this in mind, labor and delivery do not have to be scary or painful. It is possible to have a beautiful and positive experience with proper preparation and support to radiate confidence from the inside out. I'm not here to convince anyone to choose a homebirth; rather, I want to emphasize that you have **CHOICES,** starting with where and how you want to deliver your baby. You deserve to feel safe. The more stamina and low-risk you are, the more choices you will have. Close your eyes and envision your ideal birth to the smallest detail.

You know what is best for you and your family, and I'm here to support you every step of the way. Together, we can navigate this journey with compassion and expertise, ensuring you have the peace of mind and resilience you deserve. Let's connect today and start building a brighter future for you and your family!

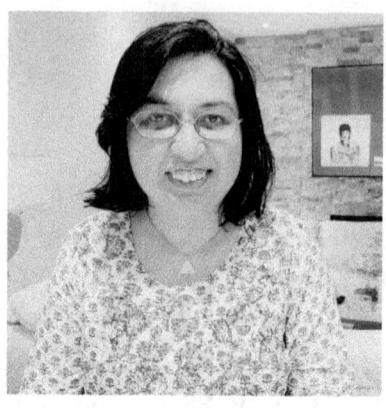

Hunyah Irfan

Founder of HunyahTravels

https://ca.linkedin.com/in/hunyah-irfan-blogger351
https://www.facebook.com/OfficialHunyahTravels/
https://www.instagram.com/officalhunyahtravels/
https://linktr.ee/Hunyah_Travels

My name is Hunyah Irfan. I'm a content creator with a community development background. I do interview of local businesses, food reviews, and travel videos. I'm also a spoken word artist. I have performed many times virtually and in person at different places. I recently was one of the influencer for Halal RibFest GTA 2024 which in my break into reviewing food festivals. I'm currently studying DBT counselling in Wilfred Laurier University.

Mental Health Wellness

By Hunyah Irfan

When it comes to mental health wellness, there are a lot of factors in taking care of health. Health can be physical, emotional, spiritual, and mental. However, mental health is where everything comes together.

If you are not relaxed at the end of the day and you have deadlines every day, then taking care of your mental health is the most important thing when it comes to your health.

These are the factors I'm going to be talking about when it comes to mental health wellness:

1. Take sleep when needed
2. Drink a lot of water
3. Healthy Living

Take Sleep When Needed

Sometimes, my morning starts at 11am. If I sleep early, then my day starts at 8am. Sleep is important to me. It helps to re-energize yourself and be ready for the day.

Some tips for sleeping:

1. If you feel drained out, then sleep in the middle of the day
2. Plan your sleeping hours
3. Sleeping early has benefits for a healthy lifestyle
4. Only stay up late when it's the weekend, not work days.

Drink a Lot of Water

Drinking a lot of water matters. When I do fasting during the fasting season, if I go a day without having water, my mind and body feel tired, and it's hard to concentrate on the daily schedule.

If you drink water, even 2 glasses a day can be good for you. Being hydrated matters when it comes to self-care. Yes, you can have Coke, coffee, and other drinks, but those are good for the time being.

However, water is something you can get anywhere and doesn't cost anything.

Keep drinking water.

Eat Fruit

Eating fruit is like drinking natural juice without making the juice through the juicer machine. Also, buying from a store is good if you want some juice or just some 7up sometimes, depending on your situation. Eating what is natural matters a lot in a healthy diet, which can be from restaurants and at home.

Eating fruits matters for many reasons.

You might already know the reasons for eating the fruits.

Try to Eat Well

Eating well matters. Not everyone, including me, eats well at times.

If there is one thing I know about weight loss, that you have to portion meals.

A bit of vegetables, rice, and meat is good, but it is important for me to reach that meal plan.

The meal plan consists of everything you need to stay healthy.

This can be vegetables, meat, rice, and salad.

It is important to have a meal in this case because it's about what you eat and how you survive. Your mental health also depends on food intake, which is how much you are consuming in a day.

That is important to know while thinking about wellness.

Stress

There are two types of stress :

1. Negative Stress
2. Positive Stress

Negative stress sometimes causes people to react. When I have too many things to do, I work remotely. Even working online can cause stress because you are sitting at the computer. Sometimes it can affect your eyesight, posture, and more.

Negative stress can be yelling and crying if something doesn't work out. For example, I sent a billion applications and I got rejected from one big project. I'm shocked. Now, that is negative stress.

Negative stress can be many things like being pressured by social groups, school and work. These three things will lead to an outcome of yelling and screaming. Being tired and not able to function properly during the day.

Positive stress occurs when you are accepted into a big project. For example, there is a back-to-school event coming up.

Then you get excited while you prepare feeling relaxed for the event. That is positive stress.

Apple Cider Vinegar

To maintain your healthy glow, drinking juice is good for you.

I recently started taking apple cider vinegar in water. This affects mental health, well-being, and overall health.

It is good for many reasons:

1. Good for mental health

2. Weight loss
3. Good digestion
4. Natural Juice you can make it at home without using a juicer

Apple Cider Vinegar balances your mental health because it is like natural juice without a juicer.

I use organic apple cider vinegar because that is healthier than synthetic apple cider vinegar.

The recommended type of apple cider vinegar is organic.

For someone like me, who gained weight during the Covid-19 lockdown, apple cider vinegar helped me lose weight. However, you do have to take it daily for this weight-loss journey.

Once a day, as it says on apple cider vinegar instructions.

This is a beneficial and easiest diet for weight loss and mental health. It also brings energy to your physical health, but it depends on what your job is.

Dark Chocolate

When trying to maintain your mental and physical health, dark chocolate is considered to be the best type of chocolate you need to eat.

There are different percentages of dark chocolate you can choose from.

Dark chocolate with 50 percent of sugar is easy to eat.

If you eat dark chocolate with 70 percent of chocolate, then chocolate is very bitter.

But this is the one chocolate that helps you with everything.

Dark chocolate is my favorite and has its benefits for many reasons.

Benefits of Dark Chocolate

1. You put into desserts
2. Good for weight loss
3. You can find it everywhere
4. Helps you with digestion

These are the factors of mental health and wellness that can be found in our daily schedule. It is all about how we react to this and that can be in many ways.

That is apple cider vinegar, dark chocolate, negative stress, and positive stress.

This depends on sleep, eating, and other things.

We don't notice it, but these are things that we should look for.

But these factors are really important for mental health.

You need to get some sleep.

You need time for yourself.

Eating and balancing your emotional, mental, spiritual health matters a lot.

Take some time to read and sometimes just take out an hour to figure out your schedule.

These things matter a lot during the day.

Remember having time for yourself is important.

This helps you plan your day and see what you need to do everyday.

I hope you enjoyed reading my take on mental health wellness.

These things are what I think matters in mental health wellness.

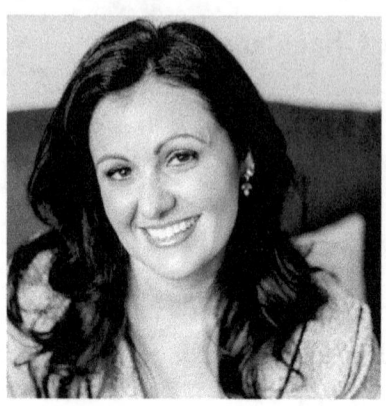

Sonia Rodrigues

Transition to Wellness
Psychotherapist & Life Transition Coach

Sonia Rodrigues has been a licensed psychotherapist for 20 years. She is the owner of a psychotherapy and coaching practice called Transition to Wellness. She has worked with people of all ages, helping them navigate various challenges in their life. She utilizes a holistic approach and provides a safe and supportive environment where her clients can feel supported on their path towards healing from their traumatic experiences and she guides them towards creating the life they desire. She provides individual therapy and coaching and also offers a variety of presentations and workshops on topics related to trauma, post-traumatic growth and fostering resilience.

Awakening Your Glow: The Synergy of Mind, Body, and Spirit

By Sonia Rodrigues

Too often, we feel bogged down by our overwhelming to-do list or depleted by the everyday challenges we face combined with the burden we carry within us of our unresolved traumas. Many of us carry burdens from these unresolved traumas that further complicate our ability to move forward, creating a cycle of stagnation and exhaustion. However, through the principles of holistic wellness, we can begin to untangle ourselves from these burdens. By nurturing our bodies, minds, and spirits, we can create space for healing and growth. When we can master the art of creating balance in our lives and healing our wounds through a mind-body wellness approach, it allows us to grow personally, professionally, and spiritually and leads us to awaken our "glow".

Holistic wellness can provide a refreshing perspective on healing and fostering growth that encourages us to delve deeper into our health and vitality. This approach encompasses the interconnectedness of the mind, body, and spirit, emphasizing that we can truly thrive when these three elements are in balance. Holistic wellness invites us to care for not only our physical bodies but also our mental and emotional well-being, as well as our spiritual essence. By embracing this comprehensive perspective, we embark on a transformative path that can significantly improve our overall quality of life.

This approach leads us to thrive and to adopt a vibrant state of being that radiates confidence, peace, joy, and an overall sense of well-being. It reflects an inner alignment and a deep sense of self-acceptance, which shines through in our interactions with the world. When we cultivate this glow, we project an energy that attracts positivity and uplifts not only ourselves but also those around us.

At the heart of this radiance lies inner strength—the resilience and confidence that come from understanding and nurturing our true selves. Inner strength is about recognizing our worth and embracing our unique journey. It is the foundation upon which our glow is built, allowing us to navigate life's challenges with grace and authenticity. As we explore the transformative power of holistic wellness in this chapter, we will explore some practical strategies for nourishing our bodies, calming our minds, and awakening our spirits, ultimately leading to a radiant glow that reflects our inner strength and vitality. Integrating holistic wellness practices and discovering how to awaken your glow from within can transform how you feel about yourself, your life, and how you engage with the world around you. Through this exploration which occurs with lots of self-reflection, you will learn to honor and nurture every aspect of your being, allowing your true radiance to shine brightly. This can occur when we let go of the burdens we carry on a daily basis by processing them and allowing ourselves to heal from them.

Many times, the vision of what we want for ourselves and our life is not what shows up, and that leaves us feeling depressed, defeated, or disappointed, but what we do not open ourselves to see is what ends up showing up for us can often be better than the life we could have imagined. Loss and change scare most of us so much that we keep ourselves from being open to the changes that life has in store for us, and this can cause us to feel stuck or keep us from accomplishing our goals. Fear and feeling uncomfortable with newness keep us in relationships and friendships that no longer suit us. I used to think I failed at my marriage because it ended in divorce, but what I learned after years of healing was that we outgrew each other, and our goals and values in our late 30s did not align with who we were when we met in our early 20s. We changed in different ways that led us to not have the same values, and when we can see the demise of a relationship as such, we see it as an opportunity for growth. When we can see this and foster that growth, we rise above the sadness, grief, loss, disappointment, and anger and propel ourselves forward to a place of growth, peace, beauty, joy, and success...a place where we can truly glow and thrive.

When we see someone who appears to have it all, we often think to ourselves, what am I doing wrong, or why can't my life look like that? At times we might even feel envious. What we often fail to see or recognize, though, is that underneath the success or the appearance of someone who has it all, is the pain and heartache that often led to the strength they currently exude and the resilience that catapulted them into this phase. I think of the Japanese concept of Kintsugi, which is the art of putting something that broke back together again in a way that makes it even more beautiful. In many ways, this can be reflective of what post-traumatic growth looks like. Who we become after we have endured our trauma, obstacles, or hardships is a beautiful reflection of the pain and suffering we have endured and how we have overcome it all.

Our glow can often arise after we have connected with our sense of purpose which develops when we have made sense of our wounds and why things have happened to us. When we can shift from the perspective that things do not happen to us but rather happen for us, then we can truly understand our journey. This concept teaches us that when certain things happen in our lives, particularly traumatic situations or hardships, it forces us to go in a different direction in our lives, one we usually do not want because it forces us to change things in our lives when we are not ready to change them, but the catalyst ultimately leads us to a more fulfilling life. In order to be open to that more fulfilling life, we need to fully heal from our trauma or significant challenges. I use the word 'trauma' very loosely because I believe we all experience some sort of trauma in our lives. Trauma includes any event that can be difficult to process or an event that has a lasting or significant impact on you.

Our healing occurs often from a mind-body perspective. Our bodies carry trauma physically and emotionally, so healing should encompass approaches that are physical and emotional, and for many, this may also include spiritual healing. Some physical and emotional approaches to healing can include yoga, meditation, stretching, all forms of exercise, journaling, practicing mindfulness, gratitude practices, and self-care practices such as getting a massage or taking vitamins, going to therapy, or doing energy work. Identifying personal strengths and areas for growth can foster confidence and resilience. Taking workshops or reading books for personal growth can also aid in healing and in feeling positive about one's life.

Practices such as mindfulness, self-care, and emotional processing allow us to confront and release the past while cultivating resilience for the future. As we embrace these holistic approaches, we can rediscover our inner strength and develop a radiant glow that reflects our renewed sense of purpose and vitality. This transformation not only liberates us from feeling overwhelmed but also empowers us to navigate life with confidence and clarity, allowing us to thrive rather than merely survive, and leading us to feel like we are truly living and growing.

Some important elements that lead to creating synergy between mind, body, and spirit include:

- **The Body-Mind-Spirit Connection**
    - Our physical health influences our mental and emotional well-being
    - Integrating spiritual practices will enhance self-awareness
    - Nourishing the body includes proper nutrition, vitamins, and hydration
    - Implementing mindful movement practices, such as yoga, dance, etc., into your daily/weekly routine
    - Focusing on sleep and relaxation techniques
    - Creating a restorative environment in your home and workplace

- **Cultivating Mental Resilience**
    - Integrating mindfulness and meditation

- Using positive self-talk and affirmations
- Crafting empowering affirmations to boost confidence
- Setting goals and intentions

- **Nurturing Your Spirit**

  - Finding your purpose through the exploration of passion and values

  - Awareness of your purpose can fuel inner strength

- **Connecting with Nature and Your Spiritual Self**

  - Exploring ways nature and outdoor activities can be very healing

  - Integrating practices for grounding and spiritual connection

- **Community and Support**

  - Build social connections in holistic wellness

  - Building a supportive network of like-minded individuals

- **Integrating Your Glow and Sustaining Your Wellness**

  - Integrate the daily practices for sustaining wellness and creating a personalized daily wellness routine

- **Celebrate Your Progress**

  - Recognizing any milestones and achievements, even small ones

  - Practicing gratitude will encourage you to look at what's going well and hopefully foster more confidence and positive growth in your life

- **Embracing Your Unique Glow**
  - o Continue exploring and nurturing your inner strength

Embracing emotional, physical and spiritual wellness is not just a pathway to healing but a transformative journey that empowers us to reclaim our inner strength and our liveliness. By recognizing the intricate connections between our mind, body, and spirit, we can effectively address the burdens of unresolved traumas that hinder our growth. As we cultivate balance and nurture every facet of our being, we unlock the potential for personal, professional and spiritual development that radiates outward, enriching our lives and leading us towards a feeling of purpose. Through self-reflection and the integration of holistic practices, we can let go of the weight and burdens we carry, leading us to achieve a more authentic existence. Ultimately, this journey towards awakening our inner glow enhances our own well-being and through our post-traumatic growth, can also inspires a ripple effect of positivity and resilience not only in ourselves but in those whose lives we also touch. By committing to this holistic approach, we allow our true selves to shine, creating a brighter future filled with a sense of peace, confidence, and profound connection with ourselves and with others.

JOIN THE MOVEMENT!
#BAUW

Becoming An Unstoppable Woman
With She Rises Studios

She Rises Studios was founded by Hanna Olivas and Adriana Luna Carlos, the mother-daughter duo, in mid-2020 as they saw a need to help empower women worldwide. They are the podcast hosts of the *She Rises Studios Podcast* and Amazon best-selling authors and motivational speakers who travel the world. Hanna and Adriana are the movement creators of #BAUW - Becoming An Unstoppable Woman: The movement has been created to universally impact women of all ages, at whatever stage of life, to overcome insecurities, and adversities, and develop an unstoppable mindset. She Rises Studios educates, celebrates, and empowers women globally.

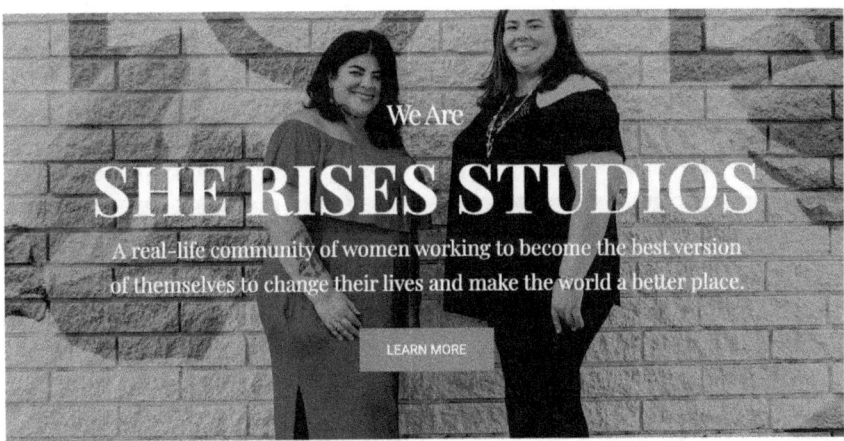

Looking to Join Us in our Next Anthology or Publish YOUR Own?

She Rises Studios Publishing offers full-service publishing, marketing, book tour, and campaign services. For more information, contact info@sherisesstudios.com

We are always looking for women who want to share their stories and expertise and feature their businesses on our podcasts, in our books, and in our magazines.

SEE WHAT WE DO

OUR PODCAST

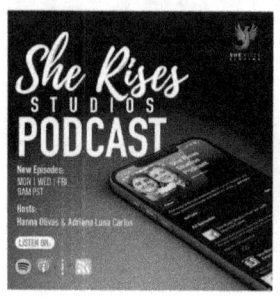

OUR BOOKS

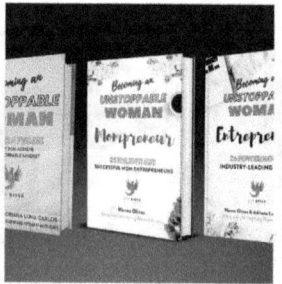

OUR SERVICES

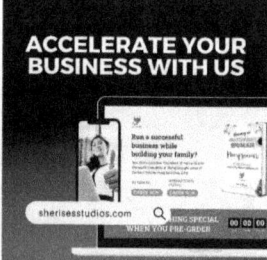

Be featured in the Becoming An Unstoppable Woman magazine, published in 13 countries and sold in all major retailers. Get the visibility you need to LEVEL UP in your business!

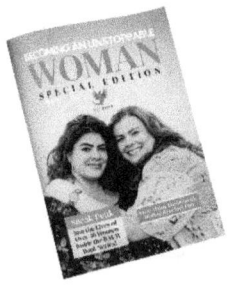 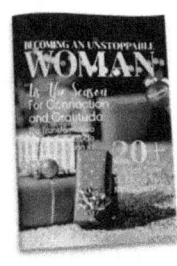 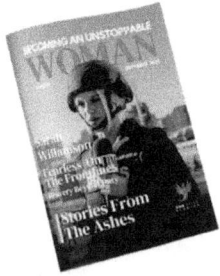

Have your own TV show streamed across major platforms like Roku TV, Amazon Fire Stick, Apple TV and more!

Learn to leverage your expertise. Build your online presence and grow your audience with FENIX TV.
https://fenixtv.sherisesstudios.com/

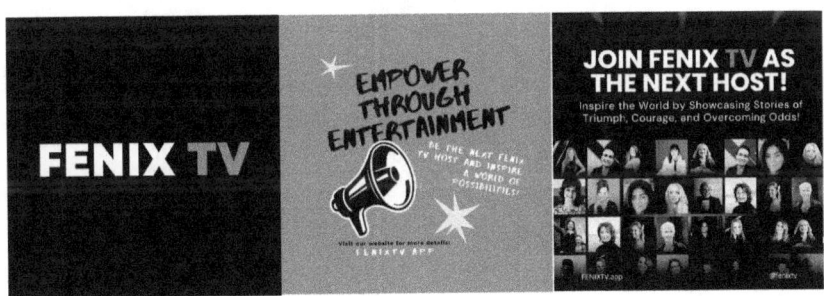

Visit www.SheRisesStudios.com to see how YOU can join the #BAUW movement and help your community to achieve the UNSTOPPABLE mindset.

Have you checked out the *She Rises Studios Podcast?*

Find us on all MAJOR platforms: Spotify, IHeartRadio, Apple Podcasts, Google Podcasts, etc.

Looking to become a sponsor or build a partnership?

Email us at info@sherisesstudios.com

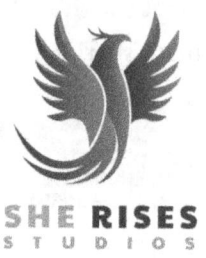

SHE RISES
STUDIOS